Hʌ

HAS

DEMENTIA

HARRY

HAS

DEMENTIA

A quest for harmonious
interaction with my
disoriented father

Dianca Schüssler

BoekenGilde | The Netherlands

Imprint

© 2022 Dianca Schüssler
Original title deMENSie (Dutch)
Translation Ton Coolen
      Karin Schüssler
      Bureau Perfect
Photo cover Lisa Schüssler

ISBN 9798224460564

Attention is the most beautiful gift one can give

Dementia is a dehumanizing condition. My father has suffered from it for many years. It pains me that he isn't always seen as a human being anymore and, at times, is even mocked. More attention should be paid to the human being behind the dementia.

As the disease progresses, I devour information from the internet, read books about dementia, and consult others who also have a loved one with dementia. Looking back, I see the mistakes I've made. I could have eased his suffering, had I been able to apply all of these lessons from the start.

In this book, I describe my own journey of discovery in dealing with my disoriented father. At the end of this book, there is a compilation of what I learned, along with the experiences of other loved ones, in the hope that caregivers will find it useful. I don't intend for this book to be pedantic. Everyone tries with the best of intentions to deal with this condition, which can be different for each person. Above all, I want everyone to have a happy, loving relationship with their loved one.

Dianca Schüssler

Content

Part 1
At Home

Avoiding the Truth

"You don't lie to your own father," I thought when my sister-in-law, who also spent years caring for her disoriented father, told me that you have to lie to people with dementia. And now I do. I lie to my father. It doesn't feel right, but I don't want to confront him with the truth. It makes him sad. In his world, he isn't ill. My challenge is to let him float around in his own foggy bubble.

Avoiding the truth is a way for me to cope. Most of the time, it's easy for me to avoid the facts. Even when he suddenly wants to go to work at the age of 72. My father retired eight years ago.

"I have to go to work," he says enthusiastically.

"Today is your day off. You don't have to go. Isn't that nice?" "Oh, is it? That's great!"

I'm not lying when I say he is off today. I'm just avoiding the truth. With time, I develop a knack for finding the sentences that work.

My mother calls.

"Your father has lost it. He doesn't remember that I have cancer, and I just tried to explain it to him. I told him the treatment will cure me. It calms him down, but by the time I crawl back into bed, he doesn't remember."

"Why tell dad that you have cancer? It makes him so sad."

"He needs to know that I'm ill. Maybe it helps to keep repeating it. It will stick at some point, I'm sure."

"I know it's a harsh thing to say, mom, but he's ill in his head. Wiring in his brain has ruptured and it's not going to heal. He freaks out the second he hears that you're incurably ill. He doesn't want to lose you."

"I know. I just can't lie to him."

"You don't have to lie. You can just avoid the truth. If you don't want to lie, just find the right words." My mother says she'll try, and later confirms that it works. He's sweet whenever she says she's tired; asks whether he can bring her a glass of water or a book and leaves her be so she can stay in bed.

Grandpa is Acting Weird

It's one summer ago and I'm staying at my parents with the kids for a week. We're in the mood for some family fun. "Grandpa Harry, let's go for a bike ride," my nine-year-old son asks.

"No, I don't feel like it," his grandfather replies.

"Let's play a game then," my twelve-year-old daughter suggests.

"Guys, Grandpa doesn't feel like it."

Disappointed, the kids grab their Nintendo and play a videogame together.

"Will you stop that racket? Go play somewhere else," my father sneers. The kids look at me, visibly startled. "Leave Grandpa be."

A bit later, they try again: "Grandpa, let's go for a bike ride and get some ice cream like we did the other day."

"No, I'm not coming. You can go without me."

My mother, who never says no to an outing with the kids, gives it a go: "Harry, why don't you go get some ice cream with the kids? They love spending time with you." My father erupts and a flood of swearing reaches the young ears of my children. "Leave Grandpa be." I comfort the kids: "I'll get some ice cream with you." We grab our bikes and head off.

"Grandpa was so mad at us."

I try to comfort them: "That wasn't very nice, was it? I guess he was just in a bad mood. It can happen to anyone." Meanwhile, I'm wondering what happened to good old Grandpa who loved to hang out with his grandkids. It dawns on me that my father's fuse has been getting shorter. At this point, I'm unaware that I will be telling my children their Grandpa is unwell in his head and will not recover.

I'm Not Crazy!

The phone rings. My father answers: "Yes doctor, I will tell her you called. Elsa has to come in for a scan on Wednesday. I'll pass it on. Have a nice day!"

At dinner time when my mother has arrived home, I ask him about it. "I heard you say on the phone this afternoon that Mom has a scan this Wednesday and you would pass on the message?" "No way. I would've told your mother." "I heard you say it too, Grandpa," my daughter tries.

"There's no way. I didn't speak to a doctor. Maybe you need to have your ears checked," my father jokingly says.

"You did say it on the phone, that Grandma has to go on Wednesday and that you would tell her," she cheekily tries once again.

"Enough! I'm not crazy, am I?" My father suddenly pushes his chair back. I try to salvage the situation: "I'm sure we just misheard." As my father walks out of the room, my daughter looks at her grandmother. "I really heard Grandpa say it." The next morning, I call the hospital. Sure enough, a scan has been scheduled for Wednesday. I give them my mother's cellphone number and have their landline number removed from the file, just to make sure no appointments will be missed.

The Businessman Fades

"Dad is being so difficult lately," I complain to my brother.

"You noticed it too, right? It seems like everything is too intense for him. I recently noticed that he knows a lot about the existing clients of our company, but nothing about the new ones. And a few weeks ago, I told him about an exciting new order we had secured. He didn't even ask once if we managed to deliver it on time. It's so unlike him," says my brother, who is now in charge of the family business.

"He forgot to tell Mom about a scheduled scan yesterday. It's as if he has dementia."

"He'd be devastated. The other day, we were talking about how our neighbor Piet is now living in an assisted living home. 'I'd rather be shot,' father said."

That night, I lie awake, unable to sleep, thinking about how odd it was that my father not asking about the big business deal. When my two brothers took over the wholesale business in brushes, painting, and cleaning supplies, my father kept a close eye on delivery of orders. This stemmed from the days when he'd drive around the country with a car full of goods, stopping at every little shop and painting company, trying to peddle his wares. Whenever his tireless efforts resulted in him securing a new customer, he treated them like royalty. This attitude turned out to be a crucial foundation for a successful continuation of the family business under his leadership. Long days were filled with hard work.

Poor souls

My father is becoming increasingly withdrawn, though I know he had the same tendency in the past as well. I remember how he would sit hidden behind a newspaper in his favorite armchair or stretched out on his reclining sofa, pretending to be asleep. Meanwhile, my mother would be busy in the kitchen, cooking and clattering with the pans. Despite leading a productive life herself, progressing from kindergarten teacher to the principal of an elementary school, domestic chores were her responsibility. Caring as she was, she didn't mind this at all. As a diligent entrepreneur, my father took good care of himself and knew how to find his moments of rest. Today, he clearly prefers to remain in the background. But at times, he still imagines himself running a bustling business. He wants to go to the shop, right now. We let him. He gets in his car, and half an hour later we greet him as he returns home. He drove around the area in a big circle but never arrived at the company.

It takes a lot of persuasion these days to get my father to go for a walk with me. He's tired, it's too cold or his leg is hurting. Many excuses this from a man who used to go on walks every day. He used to insist that we go for an hour-long walk with the whole family at least twice a week. Sometimes, my brothers and I would out of boredom rebelliously stomp around in puddles or kick chestnut shells scattered on the paths. Now, the tables have turned. And while I enjoy doing my 10,000 daily steps, I have to challenge my father to join me. Today, I succeeded with arguments like "the sun is shining" and "walking is good for your health." After a walk in the forest, we get into the car, where my father takes the seat behind the wheel. He knows the area well, but the drive is far from smooth. "We were supposed to go home, right," I suggest cautiously?

"Yeah, that's where we're going."

"I think you have missed a turn." "Come on, I know the way."

"Grandpa, the turn is definitely before that slide in that garden. I'm sure," sounds the voice of my daughter from the backseat.

"I'm not crazy! I'm perfectly able to drive home," her grandfather responds irritably. Later, over tea, my daughter sits down next to him on the couch.

"Grandpa, sometimes you forget things, don't you?"

"Yeah, old people can't remember everything."

"Does it bother you that you forget things?"

"I don't forget that much. Some people can't remember anything. Those are poor souls. Fortunately, i'm not one of those"

White lies

My mother and I gradually take on more and more of my father's duties and keep an eye on him all the time. When he leaves to get a haircut, we call the barber to let him know my father is coming. We ask him to cut him right away and explain that he has dementia. Once my father heads, home freshly trimmed, the barber calls us to let us know that he's on his way back. My mother keeps track of his agenda to make sure he doesn't forget anything, in addition to on top of taking on more and more of his personal affairs.

One day, I'm at my parents' house, helping my mother with payments. As I walk to the kitchen, my father enters the room.
"What are you doing, Elsa? What do you need that bank account for? I handle our banking affairs, you know that, right?" My father looks at her suspiciously.
"I know, but we're behind on payments and you're busy. I thought I'd help you out," my mother replies. "You stay out of it. Banking is my business." He forcefully snatches the iPad from under her nose. From now on we decide to do the financials until my father is out with his brother Jos.

The next day, my mother is about to go out for groceries. My father pulls out his wallet: "Here Elsa, is this enough to buy groceries?"

"Thank you, dear. This will do," my mother replies. "I'll have to withdraw money again," my father says.

"Shall I go with you?" I ask. My father doesn't remember the code, which is causing problems.

"No, I can do it myself," my father responds irritably. "I know you can, but have you heard about the new screens? It's harder to withdraw money for me as well, I really have to get used to it. I thought I'd help you out the first time."

"Just come with me then."

He accepts my white lie, and we withdraw the money together.

We check what my father does and make up stories. We fool him. It's a change that is especially hard on my mother. There's no room for lies in their traditional, solid marriage. We console ourselves with the thought that it's all for his own good.

Delusion

We're at the table drinking coffee.

"Did you know our neighbor is cutting down all the birches in our yard?" my father asks.

"All the birch trees in our yard? Why would he do that?" "Because firewood is valuable."

"Wouldn't he ask for our permission before cutting them down?"

"You'd think so. I'm telling you, that man is a crook."

"He always helps you clean up the driveway and the yard after a storm, and disposes of all the branches. I can't believe it."

"It's true. Believe me, he's cutting down the trees. I'm not crazy."

"Maybe you got it wrong."

"How did I get it wrong? Why does everyone think I'm getting things wrong?" My father slams his fist on the table.

"I can't imagine the neighbor doing that, show me."

We walk out into the front yard together. I don't see anything strange. My father walks back and forth in a frenzy.

"The bastard even removed all traces of felled trees. They were right here. Look, there's a heap of leaves. He did that so you can't see where the trees used to be."

"Why would he do that? No, Dad, you're wrong. The neighbor doesn't do that kind of thing. He always helps you. He's a sweetheart."

"A sweetheart? He's no sweetheart. Look what he does!"

"My father kicks a branch and walks away. "Dad, wait. Maybe you're right. Should I go talk to the neighbor?"

"Do that, and tell him to never come here again. I'll kick him off my lawn."

My father is becoming delusional. And I find that correcting him doesn't help. So, I tell him I'll talk to the neighbor, and it isn't long before we're talking about something else. We feel too embarrassed to tell the neighbor about my father's delusions.

Notes

While my mother and I rummage upstairs in her study, we're repeatedly disturbed by my annoyed father.

"Where were you guys? I've been looking all over for you."

"I told you we had to work upstairs for a while," my mother responds, agitated.

"You didn't tell me!"

"I can't do anything for myself anymore," my mother later confides in me. "He's always looking for me."

"Maybe it would help to put a note on the table," I suggest.

The next time my mother goes upstairs, she puts a note on the dining room table saying, "I'll be upstairs, in case you're looking for me." And when she goes out for a while, she writes a note: "I'm running errands. I'll be right back." The notes don't always help though. Sometimes, he doesn't see the note and she finds a confused husband when she gets back. We notice this clearly when we return from shopping together.

"Where were you guys?"

"We were just running errands."

"You could've told me that, couldn't you?"

"Look, I wrote you a note," my mother responds.

"Who writes a note? I'm not going to see that. Why don't you just tell me you're doing errands? I've been looking for you the whole time." My father roars something unintelligible and walks out. I run after him and try to reassure him.

Still, the notes often do work. To avoid writing them over and over again, we keep the scribbles in a tin.

Lost

"Have you seen my pocket comb," my father asks.

"You keep it in your inside pocket, don't you?" I reply.

"Yes, but it's not there."

"I'll help you look after breakfast."

"No, I want my pocket comb now."

"Where do you usually comb your hair?"

"Over the sink in the bathroom."

I look in the bathroom, but I don't see a comb.

"It's not there. Let's have breakfast first, shall we? Mom finished setting the table."

"No, I want my pocket comb first," my father growls.

"Let him look. He won't be eating now anyway," my mother says, taking a seat in a chair and flipping through a magazine. I can tell from her drained demeanor that she's spent many hours already searching for all sorts of things with my father. After an hour, I find his pocket comb on a side table in the room, between some picture frames. I decide to buy some extra pocket combs.

In addition to objects, my father is losing days. We buy a clearly readable clock with a day indicator and put it on the table where he reads the newspaper. We wonder if he's also losing the art of newspaper reading. Do the printed lines in the papers still reach him? He does surprise us at times, like when he walks up to me with an opened newspaper.

"Look, isn't that your house? It's in the paper."

"Let's see. Gee, you're right!"

There's an advert in the newspaper from the contractor who recently built our house. He used our house for the ad. In moments like this, I marvel at my father noticing things and remembering such things.

Acceptance is Difficult

The moments when my father is truly lucid are becoming increasingly rare. My always amiable, cheerful father appears to be slowly turning into a curmudgeon. Rationally, my mother and I know he isn't well. Yet, we linger in a phase of denial. I see a documentary on television warning about the potentially disorienting side effects of cholesterol pills. Could that be the cause? I read that a vitamin D deficiency causes forgetfulness. Is that the reason? Is it his diminished hearing that makes him disoriented and irritable? Is it due to aging, making him less tolerant and easily annoyed? We search for all sorts of excuses to avoid facing the truth. It's hard for us to accept that he has dementia in his early seventies, especially since he himself refuses to acknowledge it.

Inventing the Truth

"Watch out! You're driving too close to that cyclist!" I yell, clinging to the door.

"Not true. I know how to drive!"

My father's driving is becoming increasingly sloppy, and he often forgets the way home. He is becoming a road hazard. How do you take away someone's driving privileges when driving is what they love most? Besides many business trips, he used to drive long distances for relaxation. Our family would regularly get in the car at dusk and drive around in nature, along the winding sandy paths in the woods. The family car would burst with euphoria whenever we spotted a hare or a deer.

We dread telling him that he can no longer use the car keys. My instinct tells me we should make up an excuse. A story he'll believe, making it easier for him to accept. He receives a notification for the 75+ driving competency test.

With my father beside me, I drive to his favorite nature spot. I park the car in the parking lot. After getting out, we choose a walking path along the heath.

"Dad, you know you have to be evaluated for your driver's license renewal, right? What do you think, will you pass?"

"I've been evaluated already."

I'm not sure what to say for a moment. I decide on the spot to go along with it.

"They called mom to say you failed. She feels so bad that she can't tell you herself."

"They took my license?" he asks, startled. "Yes, dad, you're not allowed to drive anymore."

I tell him about the new policy requiring all upcoming 75-year-olds to be evaluated because children on bikes are hit on a regular basis. I make up that these collisions are almost always caused by seniors with diminished reflexes. "You don't drive as well as you used to."

"Says who? I can drive just fine. Will I get my license back?"

"No, you won't get it back."

During the walk and later over lunch, I calmly explain why he can't drive anymore. He keeps taking out his wallet, searching for his driver's license, which I've removed already. He looks at me bewildered and says, "Darn, you're right. I didn't know this morning would turn into such a bleak day for me."

Every day, for weeks on end, he keeps asking about his driver's license and his car, which we've now hidden from his view. It's difficult to watch how much pain this is causing him. And he keeps forgetting. I need to find a way to ease his pain. "Do you want to go for a drive, Dad? We'll take my car."

"No, I'll drive."

I try a different approach: "Dad, your license has expired. You're not allowed to drive. The application for a new license has been submitted."

"Oh, I let my license expire? Silly old me."

"No worries, dad. I'll pick up your license soon. Let's get in the car."

My father gets in and together we tour the landscape. He seems comfortable to accept that he can't drive his car for a while. This story feels better.

Hearing Impaired

My father and I are walking in the garden when I bring up a sensitive topic.

"Dad, I notice you don't hear very well anymore. You may benefit from hearing aids."

"I'm not going to walk around with those ugly things."

"I know what you mean, but if they helped me to hear better, I'd get them."

"I must have a cold. My hearing will be fine."

"You don't have a cold. The doctor also ruled out a blockage in your ears. We need to see a hearing specialist."

"There's no way I'm going. They just want to make money."

He is increasingly rude to my mother and accuses her of speaking too softly. The television is set to the highest volume, and he no longer really participates in conversations.

That night, I find hearing aids online that are so small, you can't see them in the ear. I decide to buy them and take them to my father on my next visit.

"What are those? I'm not going to wear those crazy things."

"Dad, listen, your friend Robert has hearing problems as well. Have you ever noticed these devices in his ears?"

"Really? Kees has them, too? I never noticed."

It works. We unwrap the earplugs together. He places them in his ear.

"It's incredible! That works really well!"

Happy and relieved, I start to chat with him. He hears everything. The same afternoon, my father grabs his ear and screams:

"I have something weird in my ear!"

And once again we explain why he has hearing aids in his ears.

"I don't need those!" he shouts.

"That would be such a waste, Dad, they cost five-hundred euros."

Since he was always mindful about money, I like to use it as a trigger now. He agrees it would be a waste of money and leaves them in his ears.

Later that afternoon, my father is sitting at the table. I close the door to the hallway. My father starts screaming and gets up wildly, "Don't slam those doors like that! It hurts my ears." He probably hasn't heard the door open and close for months. Still, I'm startled by his reaction. I've never seen him this furious before.

Every morning, my mother has to convince my father of the usefulness of the devices that go in to his ears. He's stubborn and after a while doesn't want to wear them anymore. We adjust the television settings and make sure all programs are subtitled. We buy headphones as well, so the TV doesn't have to be so loud.

Manipulation

A week before my father's birthday, he really needs some new clothes and my mother just can't seem to get him to a clothing store. I decide to give it a try. "Come on Dad, we're going for a drive. Are you coming?" I drive to the nearest town and turn my car onto the parking lot of a store.

"Why are we here?"

"Just picking something up for Mom."

"I'll stay in the car."

"I'd like you to come." My father gets out of the car and together we walk into the store.

"Look, they have nice cardigans and shirts here," I try enthusiastically.

"Don't need it."

'Well, Dad, you are wearing an old cardigan right now. Mom said you could use some new clothes. She wants to take you shopping next week."

"Shopping? I'm not going shopping. I don't need anything!"

"Grab a shirt and cardigan now, so you won't have to go next week. Mom would appreciate it. What do you think of this one?" "That one's quite nice."

"Come, let's try it on."

"I'm not trying it on."

"Well, you'll have to go shopping next week then. Better try it on now, buy the cardigan and be done with it."

My father likes the idea of being done with it now and not having to go to the store next week. We walk out with a bag full of new clothes. As I get into the car, the feeling creeps up on me that I forced him into buying things. It feels like I'm manipulating him. I console myself with the thought that he really needs new clothes. On his birthday, I hear him say that he likes the cardigan he's wearing. I don't feel guilty anymore.

Surprise Party

My father never used to miss a party. With a beer in hand and enveloped in his own cigarette smoke, he'd stand united with friends, vehemently criticizing the bureaucracy that cost him too much money. A few beers later, his loud laughter could be heard above everything else. Now, more often than not he refuses to go to parties.

My father is turning seventy-five. We notice that involving him in everything doesn't help; it makes him very restless. So, we decide not to tell him anything about our plans for his birthday and organize a surprise party.

As I drive my car into the parking lot of a party venue in the forest, my father, sitting next to me, notices family members and friends standing there.

"What's going on here? Why are there so many people? What are they all doing here?"

"It's our surprise for you, Dad. They're excited to celebrate your birthday."

"I'm not going to celebrate my birthday with them, am I?" my father responds, startled.

"Of course, you are. Look, there's David, and there's your brother

Jos with his children and grandchildren, James and Mary are also here."

"Oh, now I see." My father gets out of the car smiling. He clearly enjoys himself that afternoon.

"Your father still has his loud laugh," a relieved old friend of his says to me.

"Yes, he's still good at that, especially at his own jokes," I laugh.

"He seems very happy still."

"He is," I nod.

"But he has dementia, right?"

"That doesn't mean you can't be happy. In his world, he's still sharp as a tack."

"He forgets everything, though, right?"

"Including that fact."

"I don't notice anything weird about him."

We get the latter remark from several people that evening. It's well-intentioned, probably to comfort us. But it saddens my mother. She feels as if people are saying, "What are you talking about? Don't complain. It's not that bad."

But it's not easy at all. Caring for my father is becoming increasingly hard on my mother. I begin to notice it all the time. The saddest thing to me is that she's losing her companion with whom she shares everything. That must be such a lonely feeling.

The next morning at breakfast, my father no longer remembers there was a party. It doesn't bother us. We decide to use this trick more often. Not discussing things in advance and not telling him our plans may cause him to be overwhelmed, but at least it saves him the stress of preparation. We've been able to get my father to join many celebrations that way.

Impromptu Vacation

Even when it comes to vacations, we don't prepare my father in advance. "Where are we?"

"Don't you remember, Dad? We're going to fly. Off to Portugal."

"Oh, is that so?"

"Yes, that's right. Nice, isn't it? All of us together."

"That's nice."

"Why are we here?" asks my Dad a few minutes later.

We're watching a departing airplane through the window.

"We're about to fly to Portugal. A nice vacation together."

"Ah, yes."

The sudden confrontation works well. Seeing familiar faces in an unfamiliar environment seems to help him accept his situation. It helps that we always go to the same vacation spot in Portugal. It strikes me how he knows perfectly well where he is in the morning, and then becomes more disoriented towards the afternoon. One moment he recognizes Coelha Beach, the next he thinks he's at my house while we're actually having coffee on the terrace of a beach bar. Seeing the waves, he must realize that I can't have blue waves like that in my yard in the Netherlands. We often manage to distract him in these disoriented moments. One example is when we're at a Portuguese restaurant where he's never been before.

"I married your mother in this restaurant. Yes, yes, we had a grand wedding."

"You did. This is a beautiful restaurant. Come, let's hit the buffet again. I want some dessert. How about you?"

"I'd love some."

We're in Vienna with the whole family to celebrate my parents' fiftieth wedding anniversary. I make a booklet in advance with information about where we'll be staying and a list of things to do. I read online that this can provide people suffering from disorientation with some stability. But my father doesn't look at the booklet and doesn't want to go to Vienna. "What a waste of money," he grumbles. We put the booklet away and decide to go for the unexpected confrontation.

"Dad, are you coming? We're going out with the whole family."

"Where are we going?"

"To Vienna."

"I'm not going to Vienna. I really don't want to."

"How about we all go out for a nice dinner then?"

"I'd like that."

Half an hour later, we arrive at the airport. "What are we doing here?"

"Look, Dad, everyone's here. We're all going to Vienna."

"To Vienna?"

"Yes, isn't that nice?"

"Is everyone going? That's nice."

My father enjoys the days in Vienna.

"We got the most out of it once again," my brothers and I say to each other, satisfied, after an unforgettable weekend.

Photo Album

My father and I are flipping through the photo album from our "Together 100" party that my husband Marc and I celebrated for our 50th birthdays. I see my father standing next to my mother, smiling, and in another photo, sitting at a table with a beer in his hands, looking utterly bewildered. Seeing that picture, I remember how he sat at the front, close to me, while my husband and I fired questions at the guests. Marc and I had prepared a personal pub quiz. We asked various questions about my childhood, as well as about my past work as a manager at a secretary temp agency, and later at a large telecommunications company. After the quiz, my father came up to me.

"I didn't know you made it to manager so many times. I'm proud of you."

Later, during the dance party, he notices the photo collages on the wall and fetches me repeatedly.

"Look, Dianc, they have pictures of you on the wall. Did you know that?"

We love to browse through the album of that party or photos from our vacations together. My father often doesn't remember anything of what he sees in a picture. I'm always tempted to tell him what's in the photo. It confuses him. When I let my father browse the album at his own pace, however, he surprises me and suddenly starts to tell me what he sees. Whether it's accurate or not doesn't matter to me. He's talking and feeling heard.

Chores

"We don't need those."

"Yes, we do, Dad. Mom needs these bed risers; she's not well. She has trouble getting out of bed."

My father looks at my mother.

"Every morning, I wake up in pain and have to hoist myself up using a chair," she explains.

"Alright then, let's get to work," my father says decisively. I take the oak bed risers out of the packaging and realize they're not going to fit. Since my father is in a cooperative mood, I don't want to return them to the online store. We need to saw them to size. I persuade my father to come to the shed, where he keeps all the tools, screws, nuts, and nails, although not quite as neatly organized as they once were. I let him rummage through all his hardware, and a sense of nostalgia comes over me.

"You have such valuable tools, Dad."

"I do. Now, what was I supposed to get again?"

"A saw."

"A saw?"

"Yes, so we can cut the bed risers to size."

"Oh, right. Would this work?" My father holds up a drill.

"A great idea. But I think it would be even easier with a saw, don't you think? You're the handyman around here."

"Yes, I think so too. Where's the saw again?"

I pull out the saw from under the other tools. My father eagerly gets to work. He clamps the bed risers in a vice and saws them to size. After an hour of working in the shed, we head back to the bedroom. The bed needs to be lifted, along with the support planks. We can't lift the bed. We remove the mattresses and try to lift the bed frame but can't. Maybe we can remove the slatted frames. Still, the bed is too heavy for us to place the risers underneath. So, we proceed to completely disassemble the bed. The bedroom is a mess, with mattresses, bed planks, and two slatted frames on the floor. At first, my father is helping surprisingly well, but then his mood seems to shift.

"I give up. What a mess. Why is our entire bed in shambles?"

"We need to raise the bed. It's for Mom's comfort."

"Who came up with such a silly idea?"

"I did, she can't get out of bed in the morning. Mom's not as fit as she used to be."

"Oh. Will you clean up here?"

"I can't do it alone. I need your help. You're good at this," I say as I continue to work.

"Well, let's get on with it."

We puzzle the bed back together in half an hour. The double bed now stands on risers. Solving a problem together feels good. The mix of humor and grumbling reminds me of the father I once knew. It surprises me how well he still handles his tools. I decide to involve him in chores like this more often.

From there on in, my mother finds my father grumbling every morning, sitting on the edge of the bed, legs dangling. I can't help but laugh secretly one morning when I witness the scene.

"Why is this bed so high? Who did this? How am I supposed to put on my socks now?"

He ignores the chair my mother places by the bed for him to put on his socks, and does it sitting on the floor in front of the bed, grumbling.

We continue to encourage my father with chores. In the mornings, he feeds the chickens in the coop and checks for eggs. Next, he inspects the bird feeder to see if it needs refilling. He doesn't forget the fish in the pond either and faithfully feeds all his animals. Once he's done with his daily feeding tasks, he gets the newspaper from the mailbox.

"The lawn looks beautiful again," I say. "How do you do it?"

"Mowing the grass on time and watering it. Just paying attention to what it needs."

"It looks gorgeous. You do it well."

My father continues to mow the lawn. That green carpet is his pride. It's a win-win situation. My mother gets some time to herself, and my father is stimulated and feels useful.

Living Will

"Dad, have you ever considered a living will? It's where you outline who can make decisions about your assets and care if you become incapacitated."

"Ah, I don't need that. I'm sharp as an arrow."

"You are now. But what if you develop dementia some day?"

"We'll cross that bridge when we get there."

As I search the internet, it becomes increasingly clear to me how important this document is. Especially now that my father has dementia and my mother is ill. Someone has to protect your rights when you can no longer make decisions for yourself. If there's no appointed representative and someone is unable to manage their own financial affairs, a judge decides who will handle these matters. I shudder at the thought of a judge determining who will manage my father's affairs when my mother is perfectly capable.

I decide to try a different approach with my father:

"I was just chatting with our neighbor Anne. Her father doesn't have a living will. She has to ask permission from her uncle for things like subscribing to a newspaper for him or buying flowers for his room."

"Her uncle? You mean Wim?" I'm surprised he remembers the

name.

"Yes, that's the one. He was appointed by the magistrate. Wim isn't happy about it either. He has to keep detailed records because the magistrate can audit him."

"Piet has dementia and lives in an assisted living home, right?"

"Yes, that's right. And his children can't make any decisions for him without a judge looking over their shoulder."

"That's ridiculous. It's Piet's money, after all."

"Legally, his children aren't allowed to use it. If he had a living will, things would be different."

"A judge making decisions about Piet's money? Outrageous. What about us? Did we take care of it?"

I seize the moment and place a draft living will in front of him that I found on the internet. I walk my parents through all the decisions on financial and medical matters. They are in agreement and decide that my brothers and I will manage everything together. I go ahead and schedule an appointment with the notary right away.

Thanks to that document, my brothers and I are now legally authorized to make all decisions for our parents, should they become incapacitated, without needing to go to court.

I Want to Go Home

"I'm going home."

"Dad, this is your home."

"Don't be silly. This is our vacation home. We need to go home, and we can't leave anything behind."

My father has lived in a farmhouse with my mother for the past twenty-seven years. But it's his childhood home that he wants to return to. It's becoming a habit. Around two o'clock, he puts down his newspapers and starts pacing restlessly.

"We need to pack everything. How will we ever get all our stuff back home?" he wonders aloud, looking around in confusion.

"I'll help you tomorrow, Dad. We have plenty of time," I try to adapt to his reality.

"No, it's too much. I'll start now."

"Dad, please leave it for now. I'll rent a van tomorrow. We'll pack everything in one go. It's pointless collecting things now. We'd be doing the same work twice. Let's go for a walk together."

"A walk? With so much to do? No way!"

"Have you seen the news on TV? The Olympics are on. Let's watch the swimming event. We're in the running for some medals." I open my bag of tricks, searching for the right trigger. What worked before, might not work again. Nothing seems to calm him down, so I let him be. I watch my father walk back and forth from our house to the car, his eyes confused and his hands full of items. Once the car is full and can't fit anything else, exhaustion sets in. Only then does he settle down for tea and a biscuit, and I turn on the TV. The peaceful, pleasant hours have begun.

The afternoon restlessness is painful to watch. My father is so disoriented, and my mother doesn't know what to do. Nothing she tries seems to help. She's desperate, while getting visibly weaker and more exhausted herself. I visit the family doctor. He prescribes Risperidone, something to soothe my father's nerves. It seems to work at first, but the restlessness starts to increase again after a few weeks. Out of sheer desperation, I google: "afternoon restlessness dementia." The term "sundowning" appears on my screen. Apparently, decreasing natural light and growing shadows can trigger behavioral problems, caused by:
• lack of intense (day)light,
• fatigue,
• too many or not enough stimuli,
• irregular sleep-wake cycle.
Light therapy, good lighting, enough rest, regular meals, and a regular sleep-wake cycle might help. We agree that my father needs to spend more time in the outdoors to get more sunlight. Since my ill mother can't do it, I start going on walks with him

twice a week, his brother Jos takes him out on Fridays, and I arrange for a walking companion.

My father quickly grows fond of his walking companion. The afternoon restlessness lessens but doesn't disappear. He still tends to start packing after getting back from a walk. We try to give him his newspapers at different times in the day. In the afternoon, we offer him a freshly folded newspaper with a cup of coffee. Sometimes it works. Every day is a challenge. What will work today to prevent him from loading up the car?

Precious Conversation

"What a nice picture. You look so cute together, embracing each other in the snow like that. Why did you get married in winter?" I ask my father, pointing to their wedding picture.

"I don't know."

Our conversation isn't going very smoothly. This has been happening more often lately. I ask questions, and he gets annoyed and tells me he doesn't know and to stop asking so many questions. I see the dazed gaze in his eyes and struggle to make real contact with him.

"Mom said you went on a walk with your brother earlier."

"No, I haven't seen Jos today."

"Yes, you have. Look, here's a photo he sent me. You two had such a good time together, uncle Jos said."

"Oh, I don't remember that."

My father looks at me bewildered. I dawns on me that, despite my intentions to have a pleasant chat with my father, he is not enjoying this conversation. It confronts him with his disorientation. His short-term memory is failing. I feel foolish.

"Look at that butterfly. What kind is it again?" I try to salvage the conversation.

"A brimstone butterfly."

"Ah yes, a brimstone butterfly. What's your favorite butterfly? "I like the peacock butterfly."

"You learned to catch butterflies from uncle Hennie, right?"

"Yes, the easiest time to catch them is when their wings are closed together. You can gently grab them between your thumb and index finger without damaging the wings." "I didn't know that. And what would you do after catching one?"

"You can put it in a jar so you can see it well. Make some air holes in the lid and put a leaf on the bottom. But you have to release them soon after."

I notice that my father is proud to be able to teach me something. I realize I should talk about things that are visible and interesting to him, subjects he knows about. Another way for us to have a good time together is to look for amusing stories in the newspaper. "Read this. Someone drove their car into a supermarket."

"Sure, just park it right there."

A bit later, we're driving on a winding road passing rolling cornfields, when a carriage gets in the way. "Elsa and I got married in a carriage," he suddenly says.

"How romantic."

He looks at me, smiles, and continues, "It was a very romantic day."

"What did you like most about that day?"

"That it was over, and I could carry your mother over the threshold of our new home," he jokes.

"Gee, Dad, you really don't know how to enjoy a good party, do you?"

"Oh, I do. It was a very nice day with a reception and a wedding dinner. I just don't like being the center of attention."

The carriage in front of us makes a turn.

"Why did you choose a wedding date in the heart of winter?"

"My brother Karel would have had his birthday. It was always his special day. I wanted to keep it as a special day for the rest of my life."

I swallow: "That must've been a big loss in your life, Karel's terrible accident."

"Yes, suddenly he was gone. I felt so bad for our parents."

"It was hard for you too, Dad. How does it affect a sixteen-year-old boy to lose his older brother in an accident?"

"Yes, it was terrible. We used to sleep together in one bed."

I look beside me and see my father taking out his handkerchief to wipe his eyes.

We share a precious conversation. My father opens up about the impact of his brother's tragic accident. He tells me how fate forced him to take over the family business. And all of a sudden, he remembers why he got married in winter. He was absorbed in the moment, which is, apparently, the right time to ask deeper questions.

56

Brain Rooms

I discover that remarkable conversations occur when I join my father in the world he inhabits in that moment. Within that world, he is lucid and knows a lot. I learn to sense where his thoughts are. If I can figure that out, perhaps through a comment he makes, I can enter his world and we can have a meaningful conversation.

I come to visualize his brain as a building filled with rooms of memories. These brain rooms are precious treasures to him. They're all he has left in the final phase of his life. He lives in them and sometimes he moves to another room. Whenever I'm visiting my father, I try to figure out which room he's in. Is it his early childhood, his youth, or the space of his adult self? It's always a quest to find the open door to that room. Within the four walls of this room, I can even ask questions and get answers. I can see that when I go along with it, he feels listened to, he feels taken seriously.

My father isn't always in the mood to talk. Sometimes he isolates himself, and that's okay. Occasionally, I'm able to get his attention with a video or a photo album. Suddenly, a door to one of his rooms can open. The conversations don't have to be long. Just a few minutes can be special and so different from the times I didn't know what to talk about with him.

"Look, Dianc, that's where you got married!" My father points to Huize 't Singraven as we drive by. I'm surprised. We passed it last week and he didn't remember. I couldn't talk to him about my special day. I did not get married in the room he was in at that moment.

"I didn't know they do weddings there," he had responded then. Let's see if the room where I did get married is open now.

"What a beautiful day that was. Remember how you gave me away to Marc?"

"Of course I remember! Mom officiated your wedding. She did such a great job. And your father-in-law made a speech with great jokes."

I park my car in the parking lot in front of the house. We walk past the watermill to the restaurant. There, he points out the exact location where the wedding cake stood and where he had a laugh with my friends on the terrace.

Now I know that just because he doesn't remember something one time, it doesn't mean it's gone forever. I discover that a brain room can be closed today and wide open tomorrow.

I told a friend who is struggling to interact with his father, who has dementia, about my findings.

"Those brain rooms you told me about? It's a nice idea but it doesn't work for my father," he says a week later.

"That may be. How did you find out that it doesn't work for him?"

"I asked him if he remembered the time we won the championship. He couldn't recall that amazing day, even though I know how much it meant to him."

"Did he start talking about soccer back in the day, or did you bring it up out of the blue?"

"I brought it up. I wanted to find his soccer room."

"What might help is only asking about a topic after he's already started talking about it. That's when he's in that brain room. When you visit your father, try to figure out which room he's in first."

Two weeks later, he says: "Diane, your brain rooms idea actually works."

"That's great!"

"Yes, I was with my dad and he asked me to get a bottle of wine from the cellar. That afternoon, my father and I talked about wine for a good fifteen minutes. Turns out he still had plenty to talk about when it comes to his wine hobby. It was fun, especially since I've been getting into wine lately."

I record on the phone the conversations I have with my father. Back home, I transcribe our conversation into a document. These texts make up his life story. I document his story in a book. This sense of purpose makes it easier and much more enjoyable to chat with him. Moreover, I get to find out why he made certain choices in his life.

Frugal but Generous

"Shall we go to have lunch at Ria's bistro?" my mother asks.

"Why? We can just eat a sandwich at home," my father replies.

"And who will be preparing those sandwiches again? Let's have a nice meal out. It's lovely weather, let's go enjoy the terrace," my mother tries again. "I'm not even hungry."

"It doesn't have to be right now. Let's go around one o'clock." "Do you know how expensive that is?"

"Oh, you and your money. Shrouds have no pockets."

Money has always been a thing for my father. I try to delve deeper.

"Dad, you've always been frugal, haven't you? I actually admire that about you."

"You always have to take good care of your money, kid. You can only spend it once."

"That's true. But you also need to enjoy life."

"You can enjoy life without spending money. Sitting on my own terrace in the sun with a sandwich in my hand, looking at my garden, I enjoy it more than sitting on a terrace with lots of people."

"It's always the same with you, it can't cost anything," says my mother. She walks outside and slams the door a bit too hard. "It's always the same with her. She gets angry and walks away."

My father looks at me, puzzled.

"Mom has to cook all the time. Sometimes she just needs a break."

"Well, it does cost money."

"I don't quite get it, Dad. On the one hand, you're frugal, but on the other, you're always generous. On holidays and at family dinners, you always pull out your wallet. It doesn't matter to you how much it costs. You invested in Marc's business without wanting to see his business plan and financially assisted us with the purchase of our house."

"I want the best for my family, you know that. Besides, I want to keep something aside for when we get older, and I want to leave something for you all when we're gone."

"We need to earn our own living, you know. I'd rather you enjoy some beautiful years ahead. Why do you want to save money for later?"

"When you get older and need care, you should be able to pay for it yourself. You shouldn't burden your children with it."

I'm moved. My father has never been much of a talker. I didn't know he thought about our future that way. At the same time, I realize that my parents will probably need the money for their care sooner rather than later.

In the afternoon, we're having lunch in the sun on the terrace of Ria's bistro.

"See, Dad, it's so nice out here on this terrace. Good thing we didn't listen to you and managed to drag you along."

"What do you mean? Don't be silly. I always come with you when you ask."

I wink at my mother, who's happy that someone else is taking care of lunch for a change. I notice my mother is tired. Any energy she has left is completely consumed by caring for my father. As much as she wants to keep caring for him, the irritation is visibly building.

Help

My father can't be alone anymore in the morning. He used to keep himself busy with reading the newspapers, but it seems increasingly difficult for him to focus. He starts wandering around and opening drawers, always searching for something. My mother hires a sitter. Her free morning hours are sacred. But once she gets back, the rest of her day revolves around my father. She reassures him, patiently explains how things work, and interrupts her ironing work to check on him when she hears the front door.

My father's brother takes him out once a week. A friend of my mother's who lives nearby helps with shopping and household chores. I come to help two days a week. On other days, I call my mother. I'm blessed with flexibility as an entrepreneur, and thanks to my husband, who understands that I want to be there for my parents, I'm able to prioritize them in my schedule more and more. "Sweetheart, you're here again? Shouldn't you be at home with your kids?" My mother feels guilty.

"I've taken care of everything. I'm happy to be here for you and to accompany you on your hospital visits. I really don't mind."

I show my mother websites where others share their stories and I buy her books on dementia. I subscribe her to relevant newsletters with useful tips and advice. One of those newsletters features a recommendation by someone with dementia: "Ask one question at a time. Give me more time to find words if I need it. Don't finish my sentences for me." We resolve to be even more patient with my father.

Too Much to Handle

As I enter the living room, I hear my mother say, "No, Harry. Your mother died."

"That's not true. My mother is still alive. Just like my father. You're out of your mind."

My agitated father paces away from my mother. "What's going on?" I ask, as my mother taps her forehead with her finger.

"She says my parents are dead. That's not true. She's lying!" my father exclaims as he heads outside. I follow him and find him standing in front of the apple tree.

"Grandma used to make such delicious apple sauce."

I manage to distract my father. He starts talking about picking apples and cutting them into pieces for his mother to cook them into apple sauce with water and sugar.

"Just sit here in the sun. I'll make a pot of tea," I say, pointing him to a chair as I walk back inside. I find my mother sitting at the table.

"I just don't know anymore," she snaps when I ask why she keeps correcting my father. "He can say anything, and I just have to adapt. I'm exhausted."

My mother scares me. Her helplessness is expressed as angry shouting.

"I understand. It's hard on you. I have so much admiration for you.

You're ill and still taking such good care of Dad.

But by not going along with it, you're only making it harder for yourself. You're creating arguments you can't win."

"I know. It's so damn hard. I'm very ill, and he doesn't even realize it. He thinks I'm still his strong, healthy wife. He never asks how I'm doing."

"That's tough, Mom. I called an assisted living care service this week, they could take care of him 24 hours a day."

"There's no way. It means thath I would have people around all day. We'll manage."

"We need to prepare ourselves for when it really becomes too much to handle. Let's go take a look at that one near our house. I hear they have a good care home there," I try again.

"No, I'm not doing that! I still love your father, you know! I can't just put him away! I'll keep caring for him. Fot as long as I live."

My father doesn't realize he's ill. We decide not to have him diagnosed. The tests will only make him insecure, and there's no effective medication yet anyway. Why put him through that?

My mother and I visit the doctor. He confirms that a positive dementia test wouldn't change what care he can offer, but it's still useful to have an official diagnosis. He unexpectedly pays my father a visit and diagnoses him with dementia.

Despite my mother's resistance, I start researching home care and nursing homes.

Putting Yourself First

My father refuses to leave my mother alone, constantly following her around the house while becoming increasingly agitated and often angry at her. I buy her an e-reader and set up a Netflix subscription on her iPad. Every day, she finds a few hours for a book or a movie. Seeing her calmly seated nearby, my father settles down with his newspaper as well.

My mother has been living with a diagnosis of metastatic breast cancer for years. She says it's manageable with medication. During one of our many hospital visits, though, we learn that she needs to undergo more intense treatment.

"Now it's time to think about yourself."

"How? I want to keep caring for your father," my mother insists.

"I know, but I'm worried about you. You're getting more ill and caring for Dad is incredibly demanding. You've been doing everything for him. You need your rest. We can not allow your illness to progress, it needs to be stopped. You've done so well, Mom. I want you to stay with me for a long time."

"I am very tired, you're right about that. It's not good for my health," my mother hesitates.

"Let's take a look at the assisted living home in our

neighbourhood. We can stop by on our way home. There's a sitter with Dad now."

We visit the assisted living home. The friendly director shows us two rooms on the ground floor.
"Unfortunately, there's no availability at the moment," he says. "It's not urgent. This is just for orientation," my mother quickly responds. In the car, we both express our enthusiasm, especially for the final room we saw, with its spacious layout and private yard.

I decide to continue the search and contact several assisted living homes. Eventually, I find out there's a place available at a nursing home in the city where my father grew up and where the family business is located, about a forty-five-minute drive from my parents' house. Everything seems to come together. I persuade my mother to hand over some of my father's care, after a hospital visit reveals that her current treatment isn't effective enough. The oncologist suggests a chemotherapy with even more severe side effects.

Part 2

Assisted Living

Preparing

On Friday morning, my mother and I have an introductory meeting at the assisted living home. We enter a spacious hallway and proceed to a communal living room. We sit down at a table with the location manager. She explains that the home employs well-trained, dementia-specialized staff and volunteers. The local doctor is in close contact with the home, and there's an activities program that my father could join right away, including outdoor walks at least three times a week. She assures us that the food is fresh and of high quality.

My father's future caregiver joins us at the table. We get along immediately. She empathizes with our situation, sharing with us that her own father recently passed away from dementia, and had spent his final years in an assisted living home as well. As it turns out, my father could move in right away. I look at my mother and see tears in her eyes.

"It's so hard for this to be happening so fast. I know there's no point in delaying. I just can't take care of him anymore. I can't," she sobs.

I put my arm around her, and we both turn to the location manager.

"Don't you want to show your father the room first?" she asks.

"No, my father won't understand. I'm sure of it. What am I supposed to say? This is where you'll live? It would only cause him to panic. I think it's best to bring him here on Monday morning and stay with him for a while." My mother nods. Although I speak confidently, I don't know what's best at all. The location manager has experience with this kind of thing. Should I show him the room first?

"That's an option," says the location manager. "How do others do this?" I ask.

"It varies. We often have a prior meeting with the future resident."

"Do they understand that they'll be living here?"

"Not always. Some people come in the early stages of dementia, on their own accord."

I decide to stop asking questions. My intuition tells me we shouldn't show my father the room in advance. My mother agrees.

"Okay, see you Monday morning."

"I don't want to bring him. I can't do it. I can't leave him. It horrifies me," my mother starts to cry softly, reaching for her handkerchief.

"You've given everything, Mom. You've done so well. It's just not manageable at home anymore. Shall I bring him on Monday?" I whisper, trying to stay composed, gently rubbing her shoulders. She nods.

My mother and I walk around in my parents' house to select some furniture. She's generous and doesn't mind at all that my father will get some of their best pieces, and she is staying behind with the rest. My parents still have all the furniture they picked out together before their marriage. Surrounding my father with his own furniture might make him feel safe in his new room.

One More Family Weekend

My brothers and I take our parents to Bad Pyrmont for a family weekend - a Christmas gift to our parents, the timing of which turns out to be perfect. We stroll around the park behind the hotel where my grandparents used to spend the holidays with their children. My mother reminisces about places that trigger cherished memories of hers. My father joins in the conversation: "Remember Elsa, when we purchased that porcelain lamp from the corner shop, and I also bought a wall plate for your parents as a token of appreciation for letting me join in your vacation?"

"Yes, the wall plate. I also remember you telling a joke that made my mother really angry. She was so annoyed,'" my mother giggles. "I'm going to challenge her again with that joke," my father says, his eyes twinkling with mischief. He's in a brain room where his in-laws are still alive.

After coffee, we take my parents back to their hotel room to rest, and my brothers and I head to the pool.

Dressed and ready for dinner, we knock on my parents' hotel room door at the agreed time. My mother opens.

"Get this lunatic away from me. I can't take it anymore." She walks back into the room, crying, and collapses into a chair. Her helplessness envelopes me like a dark cloud. I enter the room and see my father sitting on the bed with a bewildered look in his eyes. "I just want to leave this place. She's stopping me. I want to go home," he shouts. Remembering a tip I read somewhere, I avoid explaining everything. Distraction helps sometimes.

"I understand you want to go home, Dad. We're hungry. Let's eat first, then we'll leave."

"I'm not going. I want to leave right now."

"We've already paid for the dinner. It would be a waste." The mention of money works once again.

"Okay, but after that, I'm going home. And she's not coming with me," he says, pointing at my mother.

"I don't even want to go with you anymore," my mother retorts.

"Quiet, Mom, stop it. He's ill in his head," I whisper to her, making sure my father can't hear.

"Yes, but I'm also ill."

"I know, but you're mentally still all here, and he's not. I know it's hard for you, but getting angry at him doesn't help. You're only making it harder for yourself," I whisper.

I help my father into his shoes and chat with him about the painting of the sheep above the hotel bed. Peace and quiet at last. As we walk to the restaurant, I realize that taking my father to the assisted living home on Monday is the right thing to do.

On Sunday afternoon, we drive back home. The movers sent us

pictures of my father's new room. My mother and I are touched by how well it's turned out. The new room captures the feel of my parents' home. The dining table they bought at an auction for their first home, which has adorned various dining rooms throughout their married life, is there with its matching chairs. Even the purple-red sleeper sofa, where my father always takes his afternoon naps, has moved to his new place.

Difficult Drive

It's Monday morning and my parents and I are having breakfast.
To my father, it seems like any ordinary morning. My mother and
I know better.

"Dad, will you come for a drive with me?" I ask.

"No, I need to read the newspapers first."

I tell him that my brother is waiting for us nearby at his company,
and that we're going to have coffee with him.

"Coffee there? Can't he come here?"

"No, he has to work at the office there and can take a break to have
a drink with us. You can read your papers in the afternoon."

"Okay, I'll come along. Are you coming too, Elsa?"

"No, I'll stay here. I'll see you soon."

Unsuspecting, my father gets into my car. My mother, clearly
emotional, stands in the doorway waving us goodbye as we drive
away.

We chat in the car about the frost on the tree branches. We pass
the canal.

"This is where I used to fish with Karel," my father says.

"Did you catch anything?" I ask in an attempt to pry the brain
room door open.

"Oh, yes. We once caught a huge carp. Right under the

overhanging branches and bushes, that's where you catch the biggest ones."

"Why there?"

"Food for the fish falls from the branches into the water - blossoms, fruits, leaves, and insects."

"Dad, we've almost reached the room we rented for you both. This way, you'll be near the hospital Mom has to go to."

"Mom is going to the hospital?" my startled father responds.

"Yes, Mom has to go to the hospital regularly for check-ups. It's convenient for you two to have a room nearby. Going back home each time is too hard for her."

"I can take her and bring her back home."

"You could, but Mom prefers to have a room here with you. It'll be okay, Dad. This will be your space until Mom improves."

"If that's what Elsa wants, I'm okay with it. She will get better, won't she?"

"They're going to take very good care of her at the hospital."

My mother and I agreed with my father's caretaker to tell him this story.

Abandonment

We arrive at the assisted living home. My brother is waiting in the parking lot. My father sees him and gets out of the car, smiling. "How nice, you're here too. Come, let's have some coffee." We ring the bell and our father's caregiver walks us down a long glass corridor that surrounds a courtyard garden. On the way to my father's room, we see some of the other residents.

My father looks at me and says, "These people are not well. You can tell."

We enter his room. It seems like my father feels right at home. He looks around and takes a seat at the dining table. My brother and I each sit on one side of him.

"Look, they've got the same furniture here as we have at home, what a coincidence," my father says. Meanwhile, he's wondering where he is exactly. My brother and I tell him this is our room. It's easier since Elsa has to go to the hospital for tests all the time.

He nods and asks, "We bought this, right?"

"Yes Dad, this apartment is ours." We avoid the truth. We're renting the room. My father hates renting. He thinks it's a waste of money. We drink coffee with my father at his new home and have lunch with him, hoping he'll feel good about the place. After lunch, my father gets up. "Let's go. I'll settle the bill."

"We've paid."

"Oh, really? I'll pay you back then."

"Don't worry about it, Dad." "Let's go."

"No, we'll stay for some more coffee."

My father always wants to pay for everything. He doesn't want to become dependent on others. He certainly doesn't want to owe anything to anyone. My brother and I suddenly realize that his wallet is particularly important to him. We decide to leave the wallet with him, and put money in it so that my father will always feel like he has enough money with him. That wallet will turn out to be of enormous value. After every meal he is offered at the nursing home, my father wants to pay for it. The caregivers respond, "It's already been paid. We enjoy having you eat with us."

We discuss with the caregiver how best to say goodbye to my father. We agree that I will try to get him to read the newspaper, and my brother and I will leave on the pretext that we have some errands to run. My father starts to read the newspaper and we put on our coats.

"Where are you going?"

"We need to do some grocery shopping."

"Will you be back soon?"

We promise him we'll be back. My brother and I leave. We close the door of his room behind us and hastily walk down the corridors of the assisted living home. "Don't think, don't think," my brother mumbles. "There is no other way, we're doing the right thing," he continues. I'm choking up.

Escaped 1

That evening, my brother calls.

"Dad escaped. I just got a call from the lady who bought Grandpa and Grandma's house. He was at the door, asking if Mom was home. Fortunately, they recognized him right away and let him in. He's there right now having tea. I'm driving up there to pick him up."

Once we arrive back at the assisted living home, my father refuses to get out of my brother's car. My brother says he needs to go in to pick up a box for my other brother, and asks if he wants to walk with him. My father agrees and willingly allows himself to be led to his room.

The daughter of another resident apologizes. "I saw your father with his coat and cap on in the hallway. He gave me a friendly nod and I thought he was a visitor. I held the door open for him." Procedures are tightened at the home. The door can no longer be opened remotely.

Meanwhile, edited photos of my father behind bars and in orange jumpsuits go back and forth in our Visit Harry family app, accompanied by comments like, "Proud of our rebellious Grandpa."

Assisted Living Proves Uncomfortable

Visits to my father are fun and stressful at the same time. How do they do things in an assisted living home? Caregivers I don't know yet, walk in and out of my father's room. Despite being friendly to all of them, my father is clearly struggling to get used to it as well. His personal caregiver tries very hard to bond with him, recognizing his sense of humor and enjoying the mischievous look in his eyes. But she has a lot to do and is going on vacation for a few days. What I'm missing most during the initial period is the sharing of experiences. What works and what doesn't when it comes to caring for my father, and can we do anything to help?

We soon notice that my father has been walking around in the same clothes for a while.

"Can't they pick up his clothes at night when he's sleeping? Back home, he used to put his clothes on the clothes rack that is now next to his bed," says my mother. "He might be sleeping in his clothes. I'll ask about it tomorrow."

"Isn't it strange that we even need to mention this? I entrust them with caring for my husband. I've known him for fifty-five years. They aren't asking any questions at all. I have brought the most precious thing in my life, not just some bag of garbage," my mother wails.

During this initial phase, I notice that the mutual expectations between the care team on the one hand, and us as loved ones on the other aren't clear. I continue feeling uncomfortable. What are we as loved ones allowed to do and what is not allowed? It feels like the caregivers have total authority over my father now that he lives in an assisted living home.

I decide to talk to a caregiver.

"Does it inconvenience you when I take my father out?" "No, quite the opposite."

"I feel like you've got complete authority over my father now. It seems like you don't encourage me to take my father out."

"We are not supposed to do that. You're paying us to take care of your father. It would be strange for me to encourage you to take care of him. But in the end, it's up to you."

From now on, I take my father out more often.

You Stink

It's Friday. I walk into my father's room and see him sitting in a chair with his back to the window. He's been wearing the same clothes all week.

"Hey, how nice. You're here too. How did you know I'm here?"

"I'm always looking for you, you know that."

"What did you bring?"

"Some delicious pastries. You get to choose first," I say and present the box of pastries to my father.

He chooses the apple pastry and eats the treat in silence. He spills a piece of pastry on his pants.

"Oh Dad, you dropped a piece. It's okay. Let's put on another pair of pants."

"No, I'll brush it away with my handkerchief."

"Dad, you've got another stain over there and your collar is dirty too. Let me help you."

"No, I don't want to!"

"Dad, you smell bad. I just want to help you."

"Really? I stink?

"Yes, and that's okay, I'll help you."

I turn on the shower. I get a clean pair of pants, a clean shirt and a cardigan from his closet. It dawns on me that this is the first time

I'm going to help my father shower and get dressed. It feels strange. He says he can undress and shower by himself, which he does. After ten minutes, I hear the shower being turned off. He comes out of the bathroom with his underpants on. I'm relieved. I've set a boundary for myself as a daughter. I don't want to see him naked. Clearly, he isn't keen on the idea either. He was always a prude. I help him get dressed. On my way out, I want to tell a caregiver that my father has showered and has changed his clothes. I don't find anyone in the hallway or the living room.

That same afternoon I send a message to the location manager: *I visited my father this morning and noticed that he's been wearing the same clothes since Monday. His shirt was extremely filthy. I know it's difficult to change his clothes, since he likes to get dressed early in the morning. Could the night shift take away his dirty clothes, so he is forced to wear a clean set the next day? I took the dirty clothes home. My mother will wash and return them tomorrow. I got him to take a shower by telling him he smells bad. It could be a good way of convincing him to take a shower.*
The location manager responds that she will make sure my father showers and changes his clothes more often.

Laundry Day

The laundry day trick proves effective.

"Harry, I need to change your clothes. Mom is doing the laundry today. You'll then have clean clothes for the week."

According to my mother, his mother was strict and he tended to listen to her. He tolerates a change of clothes more often now.

I get a call from a caregiver.

"Your father hasn't showered for a while. This morning, another caregiver and I tried to help him, but he became furious, almost wanted to hit us. He ended up chasing us out of the room."

"My father is a modest man. He hardly allows one caregiver to wash him, let alone two. You need to approach him calmly, alone, and without force. Tell him it's laundry day and his clothes smell bad. That's when he's most likely to cooperate."

My father remains upset all morning about the two women trying to undress and shower him. I ask several caregivers why they struggle to change my father. I'm surprised to find out that not all are aware of the laundry day trick.

My mother emails the location manager:

This afternoon, I visited Harry with two clean pairs of pants, cardigans, and a shirt. After chatting with my husband for an

hour or so, I suggested he put on some clean clothes. While he was changing, I noticed a bad smell. I was shocked to see his dirty underwear. There has to be a way to get him showered and freshly clothed on a regular basis. I don't mean to be difficult. I want to be honest with you. Tell me how we can keep my husband looking clean and groomed. I'm here to help.
Sincerely, Elsa

My father develops sores in his groin. My mother decides to do his laundry at home from now on, allowing her to keep an eye on how often my father's underwear is changed.

Birds

As I walk into my father's room at eleven-thirty, I'm greeted by a musty smell. I find my father, sitting in his chair with a somber stare in his eyes, unshaven and wearing his pyjamas under his clothes. His bed is not made. The curtains are half open. He looks up.

"Hey kid, it's nice you're here."

"I want to take you out today. Will you come to the garden center with me?"

"The garden center? No, I'm not going."

"I like it so much when you come with me."

"Alright then. Let's go."

"You'll have to get dressed, though."

"I am dressed."

"You are, but look, you're still wearing your pyjamas under your clothes."

"How did that happen?"

"Don't worry about it. Let me help you."

I take him to the garden center, where we have lunch and buy garden gnomes and bird food. I've installed a bird feeder from my parental home in front of his window. We return to the assisted living home, and I want to install the things we bought in his yard.

"Don't be silly. You're not putting those here. I need to take these things home."

"But this room is also our home. Shouldn't we have something nice to look at outside?"

"No, we're not putting those gnomes here."

I leave the things in the car and walk him inside.

My father grabs a newspaper and starts to read in his chair at the dining table.

"I'll get the groceries from the car."

"Thanks, dear."

I walk to the car. Grab the things we bought and carry them to the yard. I install the gnomes and fill the bird feeder with bird food. He's looking at me through the window. I smile at him. He gives me a thumbs up.

Back in his room, he looks at me smiling. "Great job."

"Doesn't it look nice? Take a seat over here, you'll have a good view of the birds."

My father walks to the sofa with the newspaper in his hand and sits down. He has a good view of the yard where a great tit just landed on the feeder. I sit down next to my Dad. Together, we watch the birds come and go. A robin arrives. We listen in awe as the bird sings an entire scale in crystal-clear notes. Our delighted eyes meet. "Did you know these little guys respond to the color red? They are known to attack hikers in the woods sometimes if they're wearing a red coat or scarf. They attack because they don't want any competition from their own species in their territory."

I laugh, "That sounds like a tall tale."

"And yet, it's true. Robins attack red. I tested it once together with Karel. I put on my mother's red rain hat when we went to the forest. After a while, I was attacked by a robin."

Challenging Stimuli

"Your father isn't getting enough stimulation at this assisted living home," my mother says with a concerned voice. "He just sits there in his chair with an absent gaze in his eyes. He's turning into a little old man right before my eyes. He doesn't get any exercise. At home at least he had to take out the trash and feed the chickens. And he used to go on walks a lot. He seems to get no exercise here at all."

"I noticed that too. Do you think he just sits in his chair for days on end?"

"I worry about it."

"He still has his newspapers?"

"Yes, but that's the problem. Nice and easy."

We subscribed my father to three newspapers at the home.

I tell the care team it's a good idea to spread them out over the day, so he has an extra moment of contact with a caregiver and a freshly folded newspaper in his hands. It used to be thought that stimulation is not important for people with dementia, but they now seem convinced that it can slow down the deterioration. As an experienced teacher, my mother knows all about the importance of challenging stimuli, and she places a plastic box full of simple children's games under my father's bed. Now we can play a game together when I'm there. My father isn't really into games, but I notice how much he enjoys it when I give him a challenge to sink his teeth into.

A caretaker confides in me: "It's so nice that we can use the games for other residents as well, but unfortunately, we lack the time."

"That's too bad."

"I agree. The games are only used for the pictures."

"For the pictures?"

"Yes, for the pictures in the newsletter for family members. So, it looks like we play games with the residents on a regular basis. In reality, it doesn't happen very often."

We commit to making sure my father gets some exercise at least several times a week. I notice that his shuffle seems to have gotten worse. After half an hour of walking, he says his upper leg hurts. At first, I can't seem to find out whether that's really the case or if it's just his way of saying he's tired. My father makes a habit of using the "leg pain" argument to end our walks. I report it to the care team. They say they'll include it in their next conversation with the doctor, but never get back to me about it.

The bare hallways in the nursing home start to bother me. There are some old history posters on the wall. That's it. Residents wander around those hallways for hours to ease the agitation they feel inside. My sense is that a hallway could be a perfect place to stimulate residents. I decide to talk to the location manager.

"That corridor is awfully bare. Can't we make it a bit nicer? I see the residents walking around there all the time."

"Well, that's what dementia does. You shouldn't excite them too much. Makes them more difficult to manage."

"That's not what I read in books and online. Maybe people thought that way fifty years ago. It's really not the case anymore."

"Well, a carnival in the hallway isn't going to give them peace of mind. Plus, I don't have the budget for it. Overstimulation agitates them."

"Too much is never good. All I mean is just a few items for the residents to experience some challenging stimuli. Like the bird feeder and the gnome in my father's courtyard. Or create a discovery corner with items from the past, which appeal to the residents."

"But the residents will walk around with these things and bring them up to their rooms."

"Have you ever tried something like this?" "No, it's not going to work."

"How about an aviary with birds in the courtyard, so the residents have something to look at. My father can feed the birds every morning."

"We don't have the time to clean the cage."

"I understand. I can do it, together with my father." "That's not going to work. What if you fall ill?"

"My brother will do it."

"And what if your father doesn't live here anymore?"

"If no other daughter or son wants to do the cleaning and you don't want the aviary anymore, we will take it home. We can put it all on paper. I saw a beautiful aviary the other day, we'd be happy to pay for it."

"No, it won't work out."

"Can I at least install a bird feeder with a gnome?"

"Go ahead."

I install the bird feeder and a gnome. The smiling gnome really cheers up the courtyard. Caregivers place chairs in the hallway, so wandering residents can take a seat and look outside.

Concerns During a Pandemic

An uninvited guest called COVID-19 enters the country. Care homes go into lockdown.

"He's only been there a month and now we're not allowed to visit him for two weeks. Soon he won't recognize us anymore," my mother sobs.

I try to reassure her, "It's not going to be that bad. It's only for two weeks. We can send him something every day, a letter, pictures, a puzzle or some flowers."

After two weeks, it turns out that the assisted living home will remain closed to visitors.

"I want to see my husband. I'm going to call the location manager," my mother roars.

"It's not her fault. She has to follow the rules set by the government."

"That may be true, but they're going to have to find a way. I see assisted living homes on TV where loved ones at least get to wave through a window. We don't even have that."

"Let's wait and see. The pandemic must be so tough on the caregivers. Let's have some cake delivered. A piece of cake for each resident and caregiver."

Two weeks later, we get the news that care homes will remain closed for at least another month.

"I see initiatives all around me. Temporary outdoor rooms being set up at care facilities so relatives can safely visit their loved ones. I spoke to our handyman. He is happy to put such a room together free of charge. I called the location manager and she says she can't allow it. "I don't understand," my mother sounds helpless.

"I'm sure she has her reasons. It would take a lot of time to get residents into a outdoor room. I've heard some caregivers have a cold and have to stay home," I try to calm her down.

"It doesn't take that much time."

"We're not in the position to judge. Hey, at least you have time to come over to our house for a while," I say, trying to cheer her up.

My mother spends days with us. A caregiver calls us regularly so my mother can talk to my father.

"Elsa, I want to come home."

"I know, Harry, but you can't."

"I have to get back to work. They're holding me here against my will."

Their phone calls are exceedingly difficult for my mother. I call the caregiver.

"Why do you let my father call my mother?"

"When your father asks me to call Elsa, for him I do it."

"But there's nothing my mother can do. These phone calls are making her very upset."

The caregivers and I agree that they won't let my father call anymore and try to distract him instead.

Meanwhile, we read in my father's care file that he's not doing well. He's wandering around aimlessly and is deteriorating rapidly. My mother sends an email to the location manager:

I don't understand why you still haven't created a safe place at the home where we can see and talk to our loved ones, especially now that Harry seems to be deteriorating. I was told that I'd be allowed to visit if he got any worse, but I fear it might be too late. I admire the fact that you keep me posted with emails and pictures, but it would mean so much if I could just spend some time with him.

Window Visit

It's now two weeks later and my mother and I are standing awkwardly outside, in front of the window to my father's room. He sees us, and a faint smile appears on his lips. We're seeing him for the first time after six weeks of not being allowed to visit. We can see he's saying something, but we can't hear him. The windows are shut. The caregiver yells, "Your father says 'why are you standing out there? Come in!'"

"We can't, Dad. COVID."

"What are you saying? I can't hear you. Come inside!"

"We can't. COVID. You know, the virus." The caregiver explains to him what we're saying.

"Don't be ridiculous! Just come inside!" He walks towards the window and tries to open it, but the caregiver stops him. I came prepared and brought my father's old cellphone. I desinfect it and pass it through the now-opened window to the caregiver, who then closes the window again. I call my father. The caregiver helps him answer. My father doesn't understand. He storms out of the room, shouting, "I'll let you in!" The caregiver follows him. Moments later, my father reappears at the door with the caregiver, she's holding a cup in her hands.

"Sit down, Harry. I've got a cup of coffee for you."

"They need coffee too," my father says, pointing at us. "It's not allowed."

"Why not?"

"It's okay, Dad. Mom and I just had coffee. We're just happy to see you."

"Come again? I can't hear you!"

"We're really glad to see you!"

"What?" My father can't hear me. His dejection is visible.

My mother whispers, "Oh my, he's crying."

Our first window visit is not a success. The problems posed by a closed window had not been considered.

"A baby monitor isn't that expensive. They could even get one on the internet," my mother and I agree in the car on the way home. Overwhelmed by the sad situation we've found ourselves in, we spend the remainder of the ride home in silence.

Powerlessness

No working baby monitor is provided. The window visits aren't working for us like this. They only makes my father restless. After three window visits, we decide to stop.

We are desperate and are considering ways of having my father move back home again. We are in tremendous doubt. It seems like my father just got used to being in an assisted living home. What are we doing to him? My mother sends an email asking if it would be possible to have my father move back home for a while. The location manager responds:

It's possible if both doctors agree. I don't think it would be a problem in this case, since he has only just been deregistered from your old doctor. Of course, we have to be sure that he doesn't have COVID. Do keep in mind that if he gets ill and you need help (home care, for example), it' will be nearly impossible to arrange that in the present curcumstances. Harry can return to us when the government measures are over; when the assisted living home is reopened for visitors.

My mother emails back:
It's very difficult for me to deal with the fact that the doors of the assisted living home will remain closed until May 20th. It

saddens me a lot. You're aware of my doubts about leaving Harry with you during these times. I know you take good care of him, but he's also clearly deteriorating. It's unbearable for me to not be able to be with him. It's a terrible dilemma. But for now, we've decided to leave Harry in your care.

After May 20th, the COVID rules are relaxed nationwide. For the first time, my mother is allowed to visit my father in a separate room with only a table and two chairs. Afterwards, she writes this emotional email to the location manager:

I was with Harry this morning. It was a pleasant hour. Harry didn't like the space we were in and wanted us to be together in his apartment. I couldn't agree more. He clearly loved the time we had together. And a great sadness came over him when he was taken back to his room. He wanted to say goodbye to me the way we always do. He got up, wanted to walk towards me, and was pulled away by the caregiver because of COVID. The intensely sad look I got from Harry is etched in my mind. I want this to change. This is not okay. I was tested for COVID at the hospital last week due to the 1,2 liters of fluid that had to be pumped out of my left lung. I tested negative. In addition, I've been in quarantine continuously due to my illness. I urgently ask you to please find a decent solution for the both of us, Harry and myself.

Kind regards, Elsa

The location manager responds by email:

Dear Elsa,

It's nice to hear that you had a quality hour together. We've got an hour available this Wednesday, should I schedule you in for an extra visit?

I understand that it'd be even more comfortable in his room. Unfortunately, we can't allow it just yet. The reason is that visitors would have to walk through the assisted living home, which is impossible without encountering the residents. Plus, the apartment has to be cleaned after every visit, which is a lot more convenient in an apartment that isn't fully decorated. However, since you tested negative for COVID, we can make an exception for your goodbye moment. As far as I'm concerned, it's okay for you to touch each other (while wearing a mask, of course).

A week later, the COVID rules are relaxed even more, and I'm allowed to visit my father in his own room.

"Isn't it nice for me to be here again." "Take off that silly thing."

"It's a mask, I have to wear it."

"Come again?"

"Dad, I have to wear it due to COVID. You know, the virus that's been ravaging the world. The government has mandated these masks."

"I don't care about the government. Take that thing off."

Every visit I'm required to wear a mask in my father's room, this medical travesty is the subject of our conversation. It just doesn't get through to him that I have to wear it. Normally, I always look forward to seeing him, but now I'm starting to dread it. I can see the frustration caused by the mask.

I notice that decisions are being made by people who have no idea of what it's like to have a husband or parent in an assisted living home during COVID. My father finds it difficult to understand me when I wear a mask. I think it would be perfectly safe for me to visit my father without a mask, provided I have a negative test and keep my distance. I talk to the loved ones of other residents, and they feel the same way. I decide to join the central client council of the overarching national care institution. I don't want to feel this powerless anymore.

My father hasn't been outside for three months now and lost twenty pounds during that first COVID wave. Once I'm allowed to take him out for a walk again, I'm shocked to see my father in such a bad state and walking with such difficulty. My brothers, uncle and I take my father for a walk outside every time we visit. It strikes us how quickly his walking improves. His muscles gain strength and his smile returns.

Sharing the Care

Even though the COVID rules have been relaxed, healthcare during the pandemic proves to be a challenging profession. I watch the caregivers go from one resident to the next, clearly short on time.

"Communicate with me!" I keep saying, "How can I help the care team?" I ask repeatedly.

"My feet hurt so much," says my father, as we return from a walk. "Where does it hurt?"

"Here." My father points to the tip of his shoe. "Let's take a look." I roll down his socks and nearly throw up at the sight of his dry feet with twisted and bent toenails, so long they almost pierce through his shoes. "No wonder it hurts, Dad. I'm going to trim your nails." I trim his nails and rub his feet with heavy cream. After taking care of his feet, I give him clean socks. As I tie his shoelaces, I hear my father say, "This is so nice. Thank you."

On another visit, I notice him rubbing his hand on his groin.

"It hurts so much right here."

"Let me take a look."

Despite his shyness, he allows me to take off his pants. His underwear is soaked with urine, and he's probably been wearing it for days. Just underneath his underwear, I notice a red sore spot in his groin. I confront someone from the care team. "I know you're all very busy and my father can be stubborn. But this is really shocking."

"I completely understand. This is horrible. Your father doesn't want to shower at all lately."

"Why didn't you tell me? I could have tried."

"Yes, I'm sorry. I'll pass on the message that we need to try showering him more often."

"How is that message passed on?"

"In the care file."

"Do all the caregivers read the care file?"

"Not always."

"So, what's the point of putting this information in the care file? Wouldn't it be better to put up a note or a care schedule in his room?"

"Yes, that would be better. But the location manager is against it."

"How do you ensure that if my father refuses care, it will still be provided later?"

"We don't, or we just tell each other."

"You mentioned earlier that you hardly have any time for handovers?"

"Yes, that's true. Things are not well organized around here. I'll make sure to check that your father is being washed."

"That's kind of you. And please check his shirt as well. I always find a thick black rim in his collar."

"I'm really sorry about how things are done around here. I promise to keep an eye on it myself."

After that incident, I try to shower my father every time I'm there. Often, I succeed. The caregivers and I praise each other when we manage to get him in the shower. Fortunately, he can still put on his underwear by himself.

I'm at a play about dementia that is also attended by caregivers. The actors joke and make light of loved ones who complain.

"Does this ring a bell? Just when you're extremely busy, some family member comes over to complain about untrimmed toenails."

That comment stings.

Escaped 2

We're on a family vacation in southern France. I'm strolling along the boulevard of Mimizan when I'm startled by the ringing of my phone. As I open my handbag, the screen of my cellphone tells me it's my mother.

"Your father's gone," she sobs.

"What? Dad died?" A sense of fear wraps around my heart.

"No, he escaped and he's wandering around town somewhere. I know there's nothing you can do right now, but I just need to talk to someone. He's in serious danger, with all those big roads in the city." My mother is freaking out.

"But Mom, do they know where he is?"

"Yes, a caregiver is following him around, but he seems to be quite angry with her."

"Oh, so someone is keeping an eye on him. I'm sure it'll be okay.

My brother who was called into action, tells me later that my father walked for an hour with just one goal in mind: to get back home. In the end, my brother picked up my father and his caregiver at my father's childhood home. The caregiver had a sense of humor about it, despite being exhausted. Especially since that morning, she had decided to wear flip-flops to work, because of the heat.

"I'm never doing that again," she assured my brother later over coffee.

Client Council

I join the central client council of the nursing home's overarching care organization and design a COVID survey. I want to understand how other families experienced the COVID period, and they share familiar stories. Together with four other members, I establish a focus group within our nursing home.

Various pain points emerge from the first focus group meeting:

"I want to talk about the care and the caregivers. They are trying to provide good care but can't manage it due to lack of time. They have far too little time for handovers. I visited my aunt recently, and she was still in bed in her pajamas. It was two in the afternoon," says a caring niece.

"I want to talk about how the residents don't get any exercise. My mother hasn't been outside for the entire duration of the pandemic, even though she loves to go for a walk. Do they even have an activities program at all? I asked the location manager about it recently but am still waiting for a response. Plus, my mother received the wrong medication last week," a worried daughter shares.

Another daughter expresses her dissatisfaction, "That's a big problem. I've never seen an activities schedule either. Activities don't have to be difficult. If residents want to help with household chores, let them. Let them do laundry and ironing or take out the garbage. This is their home. It's not a hotel. Let them do things they used to do at home. Though, it really feels like a hotel, with those cold, empty hallways. And nothing ever goes on there."

"I've discussed this with the location manager. She doesn't want a circus in the hallway. Residents get too agitated from all those stimulating activities, she says."

"Where does that come from? That's not true at all. They shouldn't be overstimulated, but they need some stimulation. Read a book on dementia and you'll know."

"I want to talk about clothing. My father's closet is a mess. And I always find other residents' clothes there. Plus, my father's room isn't cleaned properly. I'm embarrassed when he has visitors. It's terrible that I have to clean it myself when I know someone's coming," says a concerned daughter.

"Did you know they clean your father's room on Friday because they know you're coming on Saturday?"

"Is that so?"

"That's what one of the caregivers told me the other day. She says it's a disgrace. There's a culture of keeping up appearances here."

"That's outrageous. We're being deceived while paying top dollar for this home."

"I brought my father to the living room around dinner time the other day and saw they were putting meal plates in the microwave.

We chose this home because their website says they prepare fresh meals, which isn't true."

We decide to schedule a meeting between the location manager and the focus group.

Meanwhile, I continue to contribute to the central client council. I critically assess consent documents about food, drink and housing, and a fellow council member and I write up job profiles for a regional manager and a location manager. For the latter, I include the requirement of being a warm, motherly figure.

The focus group meeting with the location manager goes well. We're able to discuss all the agenda items. The location manager promises improvement. The caregivers are informed and say they are especially pleased to have more time for handovers. They like the idea of involving residents in daily chores. The caregiver now takes my father outside to take out the garbage. A few days later, I read in his care file that he's been grumbling while sweeping the leaves. It makes me laugh and cheers me up, just like it used to at home.

Unfortunately, the improvements are short-lived. Two good staff members leave the care team. The caregivers indicate they no longer have time for proper handovers and extra care for residents. I escalate the issue to the director. An online meeting follows between the regional manager, the location manager, and the focus group members. Hardly anything changes.

Reward

The second wave of the pandemic arrives, bringing with it a renewed mandate for mask-wearing at the assisted living home. I am allowed to visit my father in his room for an hour, but I have to keep my mask on, and we're not allowed to have coffee. My father is furious when I don't remove my mask. I approach the location manager, requesting an exception because visiting my father under these conditions isn't working at all. My request is denied. I call the chair of the client council and members of the COVID team.

Later that day, I get a response from the chair:
"I've got some good news for you. The COVID team understands your situation, and the rule will be relaxed across all facilities. You can drink coffee with your relative in their room without wearing a mask, provided you stay seated at a distance."
Elated, I call my mother: "Mom, we can have coffee with Dad again."
"Really? It's allowed? Even the location manager is okay with it?"
"Yes, Mom, she has to comply. It's now a nationwide relaxation of the rules in all assisted living homes."
"That's wonderful," my mother responds, audibly emotional. My

joining the central client council hasn't been in vain.

The caregivers are denied a budget for decorating the hallway, despite multiple requests to the location manager. As the relatives of their residents, we appreciate their dedicated care. We gift the caregivers a digital photo frame filled with engaging pictures for the residents and two display cabinets to showcase recognizable items from the past. The caregivers assemble the display cabinets with the help of a resident. Now, residents wandering around those long corridors will sometimes pause to look at digital photos or old model cars in a display cabinet.

In one of the client council meetings, I learn that each home will receive a quality budget for hiring an activities coordinator who will develop and oversee an activities program. Additionally, I secure a budget to fulfill the wish of the caregivers at our assisted living home: a laundry service with a staff member dedicated to handling the laundry. Being a member of the client council of your relative's assisted living home truly pays off.

Bucket Full of Tears

My mother is dying and has now become a resident of the assisted living home. My father's kind caregiver arranges for her to spend her final days in the room next to his. Since the pandemic is still raging, the location manager only allows two people at a time in my mother's room, despite her having three children. She catches us as we walk into my mother's room and sees me in the kitchenette while both my brothers are at my mother's deathbed.

"You come with me," she screams at me.

I nearly drop a cup on the floor and follow her into the hallway, closing the door to my mother's room behind me.

"How many times do I have to tell you? Not all three at once," she yells. "I'm sorry. I know. My brothers came unexpectedly. That's why I went into the kitchenette. Everyone sanitized their hands. We're all wearing masks and keeping distance."

"It's not enough. We had an agreement about this. Make sure one of you leaves right now," the location manager snaps at me, continuing down the hallway as I shakily open the door to my mother's room.

"Don't let her get to you. Look how she's treating you. It's not right," my brother rages, after apparently overhearing the whole thing.

"She has no right to lash out at you like that. After everything you've done for this home," my mother whispers with a fragile voice.

"Calm down, Mom. It'll be okay."

"No, it won't be okay. Your father is still here. They need to pay more attention to how these people are cared for. She's responsible and she's not doing a good job."

"I know, Mom. I promise I'll take good care of Dad."

My brothers leave. I sit down beside the bed and watch my mother fall asleep. I look at her sunken face, pained that she had to witness such an outburst. Despite her illness, she's gone above and beyond to care for my father as best as she could. I deeply respect the way she carried her illness.

"A bucket full of tears is useless. It won't help," she'd say after yet another bad test result, and sure enough, we'd end up enjoying pastries and having a laugh. I happily drove to my parents' house every two weeks, and we talked on the phone every day. We were sad, of course, but we also had a great time together. My mother was always busy making plans, such as organizing a party for the holidays or making a digital photo frame for the nursing home. I would help her with a smile on my face. We were both so happy to have a purpose. It dawns on me that I'm about to lose her. My mother wakes up, sees the tears in my eyes, strokes my hand and says, "Never forget, there's always a ray of sunshine somewhere."

Farewell

The care team at the nursing home is visibly struggling with the challenges brought on by the pandemic. Meanwhile, the true heroes of the healthcare system show their strength. They push the boundaries of the pandemic regulations. They understand the pain of not being allowed to sit beside your dying mother in her final days.

They whisper, "Go in through the back door to your mother's room. I'll leave it open for you, so all three of you can be with her." Or, "Just take off that mask. Give her a hug. Hold her while you still can."

These healthcare heroes risk their own positions and trust the common sense of the residents loved ones. It seems absurd that any newly recruited intern can hug my mother, but her own daughter has to keep a distance.

My mother's alarm button is malfunctioning. The caregivers say these buttons break all the time and they inform the location manager. As a precaution, she's given three alarm buttons.

"Why so many?" I ask.

"Just in case. They operate on Wi-Fi and batteries. You never know." I go home with a heavy heart. It's the night before the day my mother will pass away. In the middle of the night, she calls me in a panic.

"I need to use the bathroom and none of the alarm buttons are working," she sobs.

I immediately call the nursing home and, to my relief, get through to the caregiver on night duty. She's alarmed and rushes to my mother's aid.

The next morning, after speaking with the doctor, and it becomes clear that my mother is dying, I'm sitting by her deathbed with my father. He has a moment of clarity.

"Are you very ill, Elsa?"

"Yes, Harry, I'm very ill. I can't go on." My mother takes my father's hand.

"Oh, what a pity. I love you," my father sobs, wiping away a tear with his handkerchief.

"I love you too, very much. I would relive our years together in a heartbeat."

"Me too. They were some beautiful years."

"Very rich years."

Watching my father gently embrace his weakened wife, I'm overcome with emotion. I gasp for air and quietly step out into the hallway.

An hour later, my brothers arrive. The location manager makes an exception and allows all four of us to be with our mother, despite the pandemic regulations. We share one final warm, intimate family moment together. My father becomes visibly tired. My brothers take him back to his room, where he no longer recalls that his wife is about to die.

Thanks to my fathers caregiver, we're able to say as children a dignified farewell to our mother, our greatest supporter.

Human

After my mother's passing, I find myself in the service room across from the location manager.

"You yelled at me while my mother was dying, and she could hear the whole thing. I was really hurt by that."

"I have to make sure that pandemic measures are implemented," the location manager says in her defense.

"We had just one person to many in the room, I regret that, but you could've handled it differently. The way you spoke to me is unacceptable."

"But I'm charged with ensuring that everyone adheres to the rules."

"You're enforcing these pandemic regulations to an inhumane degree. Some caregivers ignore the rules at times in order to make things more humane around here, without ever compromising safety. They exude warmth and trust. I feel like you don't trust me."

"I do trust you. But headquarters expects me to follow the rules. That's what they expect from a manager."

"You can be flexible about certain rules. Like the time my mother showed up on your doorstep with an urgent need to go to the bathroom, and you refused to let her in, suggesting she go to a gas station. You knew she was in strict quarantine. That's what I mean by being inhumanely strict and lacking trust."

"I did let her use the bathroom."

"Only after she burst into tears. A location manager should stand up for caregivers, residents, and family members. I don't see that in you. I expect a location manager to be the nurturing mother of the assisted living home."

"I used to be a warm person before the pandemic," she says, visibly upset. Her eyes tear up and I sense the helplessness and emotions in the dilemma she faces.

"I can see that you work hard. Whenever a caregiver is sick, you take their shift. I admire you fore that. You're doing your best," I try to console her.

"I am. Headquarters is very demanding. I will try to be more humane about the rules."

I discuss the events of my mother's passing in the monthly client council meeting. "I feel like such a complainer. Every meeting I bring up something new."

"You shouldn't call yourself a complainer. You're a positive improver. We're concerned about the lack of improvements at the assisted living home. These emergency buttons weren't working even before your father moved in."

The client council president sends an urgent letter to management about the malfunctioning emergency buttons. The assisted living home gets a new alarm system.

Funeral

We're sitting on a wooden bench at the front of the church, my brothers, my father, and I. Next to us, the coffin with my mother, covered with a floral masterpiece. Due to the pandemic, there's a maximum of fifty attendees to the farewell service. My father looks around and nudges me.

"Whoever is in that coffin wasn't exactly popular. There's almost nobody here."

I try, yet again, to explain the fact that there's a virus going around, that's why the funeral is so small, and it's also why we're all wearing masks. Initially, my father refused to wear one.

"COVID? Never heard of it."

"Dad, please. Everyone is wearing a mask. The Minister of Health says it's necessary." He agrees, reluctantly.

"Who's in the coffin?" my father asks as he rocks back and forth on the church bench.

"Dad, don't you remember? Mom was ill and passed away peacefully."

"I didn't get to say goodbye," it echoes through the church.

"You did, Dad, and you did it well," I whisper. "Remember sitting beside her bed, taking her hand, talking about how much you love each other and the beautiful life you shared?"

My father gazes into the distance, dabbing his teary eyes with a handkerchief. His gaze shifts from the altar to the coffin, then he turns around, smiles at some acquaintances, and nudges me again. "Who's in the coffin?"

Alive and Well

I visit my father the day after the funeral. "It's so nice you're here. Your mother will be pleased. She's getting groceries."

"A necessary chore. Look, I brought flowers."

"They're beautiful. Elsa will be pleased." I go along with it, he's so cheerful.

My brothers and I decide to keep up the illusion that my mother is still alive. The location manager disagrees at first and suggests making a photo album with pictures of my mother's deathbed and funeral so they can explain her passing to my father. She even suggests putting a photo on his nightstand, of my father next to the open coffin, to remind him that his wife has died. I don't like the idea; why would we make my father live through the sorrow over and over again? I even regret taking him to the funeral. Why did we do it? Was it for ourselves? For the sake of appearances? Because my mother would've wanted it? It only brought him a great deal of pain that day. The image of my father crying as he walks behind the coffin is etched in my memory. Mourning takes time. And time is something he doesn't have because he keeps forgetting. As soon I tell him once again, the mourning process starts all over. How do I convince the location manager of the assisted living home that we shouldn't be confronting my father with the passing of his wife all the time?

Suddenly, I recall the dementia coach I met a year and a half ago during her presentation, "Attention for Dementia." I was impressed with her approach. That night, everything I'had experienced and felt in dealing with my father fell into place. I decide to get in touch with her.

"Your father lives in a world where your mother is still alive," she says. "Why would you want to hurt him by telling him that his wife has died over and over again? Just go along with it."

The caretakers tell me that my father is satisfied with the following answer to his question.

"Have you seen Elsa around?"

"No, not today."

"She should be here soon. She knows I'm here, right?"

"Yes, she likes you being here."

It works. My father is happy every day. In his world, his sweet Elsa is still alive and well.

We replace my mother's funeral card on the cabinet in his room with a cheerful black-and-white picture of my young parents dancing with each other. I tell the care team the story of how my father asked my mother out to a dance fifty-six years ago. My father told me the story as well. He beams when he recalls these love-filled memories. Now that the caregivers know the story behind the photo on his cabinet, they will sometimes grab the picture and ask my father about it. Sometimes, his brain room is closed and he doesn't remember. But when the door to that room is open, my father will enthusiastically share his story.

Moving

I feel no warmth at my father's nursing home. Some good caregivers have accepted jobs elsewhere. Even though there is now an activities coordinator and a laundry service, my father still smells bad and walks around with a beard under his chin; this is a man who always hated having a beard. I clean his room every time and check if any of his clothes need to be changed. On top of that, the staff rarely undertake anything with my father. The promises made at the intake about fresh food and an activities program have not been fulfilled. The relationship with the location manager is fine, though I find it hard to accept her often harsh actions. I realize I'm not going to change that. While I'm not looking forward to saying goodbye to my father's kind caregivers, but my intuition is screaming at me to get him out of there.

I'm offered a room at another nursing home, where I had a viewing with my mother a year and a half earlier. She stood in the room and looked out the window into the courtyard, where she saw a bird feeder. She sighed:

"This would be a wonderful place for Harry."

There was no room at the time. There is space now, and it's that exact room. We make a difficult decision. We're moving my father on his birthday. It's almost like someone, looking down on us, arranged it.

I say goodbye to the client council and conduct two exit interviews: one with the chair of the client council and one with the new director of the care organization in question. I tell them that leaving is the only option when you realize that no matter how hard you try, there is no short-term improvement for the people who live and work there. My father doesn't have the time to wait for improvements promised in the long run. I keep reading how poorly people with dementia deal with moving. To make the move as smooth as possible, his brother Jos picks up my father for an outing.

During the move, we find two large cabinets and a table in his room that do not belong to him. The caregivers don't like it, but we move the large cabinet and table to the common area of the assisted living home, the conservatory. He wouldn't recognize that furniture. The closet, however, is too big to take apart. We have his old closet in the moving truck. We take the easy way out and leave the other one behind. To this day, I regret it. Every time we're about to go for a walk and I want to get his coat, he says, "You can't go in there. That's not our closet."
It also keeps breaking. We've spent a small fortune fixing it. Unfortunately, we don't have his own closet anymore.

When my father arrives at his new room, all his furniture has been installed and his paintings put up on the wall. "Hey, all my stuff is here."

"Isn't that great? Here's your chair, where you like to read your paper."

My father adjusts quite easily. I hand out and email a document to the new care team, describing in detail everything I want them to know about my father. It covers the following topics:

- character traits and hobbies;
- his married life, the death of his wife and how we deal with it;
- his hearing impairment and why he fears doctors;
- why carrying a wallet is important;
- tips to make his daily care run smoothly;
- TV programs he enjoys watching;
- what he likes to eat and drink;
- topics of conversation that appeal to him and that he knows a lot about;
- his need for some encouragement in social interactions.

Being a Carefree Daughter

On the very first day, I have a conversation with the caregiver at the new assisted living home.

"I hope we can meet your expectations." "No need to worry. We're just looking for a caring environment. We're not an annoying family with excessive expectations. All we want is for him to look like he's being cared for, that he's washed and shaved daily and wears clean underwear, that his clothes are changed every other day."

"That goes without saying."

"Well, it turns out that not every assisted living home sees it that way. Though I do realize my father can be quite difficult at times."

"We're happy to accept that challenge. Also, I think the dose of your father's medication is very high. I've made an appointment with the doctor who comes here weekly."

"Dose too high?"

"Yes, way too high. Higher than any other resident here. Were you in contact with the doctor at the previous nursing home?"

"No."

"We think it's important for the doctor to know our residents. The doctor visits every Tuesday."

I open the front door of my father's new assisted living home with the key I was handed personally. I no longer have to ring the doorbell and wait for a caregiver to open the door and walk with me. With a full basket of nail clippers, cleaning wipes, a fresh bunch of flowers, magazines, fruit and a box of pastries in my hands, I walk into my father's room.

"Hi Dad, don't be alarmed. It's me, Dianca. You look like you're enjoying that paper."

"You're here? How did you know I'm here?"

"I keep an eye on you," I smile.

"Well, nice to have you here. I love those flowers. Elsa will be pleased."

"Yes, I bought them for you. I'll put them in a vase."

"Do you have enough money to pay for it? Your allowance isn't enough for that. I'll pay you back for the flowers."

"Don't worry about it. It's my treat. It smells so nice in here."

I look around and notice how clean the room is. I can hardly believe it as I drag my index finger across his closet. The cleaning wipes can stay in my basket. I last trimmed his toenails a few weeks ago. It's time. I take the nail clippers out of my basket.

"Let me take off your shoes, so I can trim your nails."

"Why would you cut my nails? I can do it myself."

"I know, but you don't have a good clipper here. So, I brought my own. I thought I'd trim your nails this time, and if you like this clipper, I'll buy you the same one."

"Why doesn't Elsa buy a good clipper?"

They were sold out. Mom knows I trim your nails now. She likes it."

"Oh, okay."

My father lets me take off his shoes. I let his socks slide off his feet. I see well-groomed feet with clipped nails. It moves me. A caregiver walks in as I'm tying his shoelaces. She's carrying a tray of fruit for my father. "How lovely, you have visitors. Can I bring you coffee or would you like some fruit, too?"

"I can make the coffee myself."

"Don't worry about it. Sit back and relax. You enjoy your time with Dad." His clothes are washed and ironed every day. His closet is organized. His bed is neatly made, though it does strike me how narrow it is.

I meet the activities supervisor in the first week.

"What does your father like to do?"

"He likes to take walks."

"Well then, we'll be taking him around on a regular basis. We can also go on bicycle rides with our tandem bike."

"I think he'd like that. At the previous assisted living home, they'd rarely take him out. We made a walking schedule for him ourselves. We'd pick him up three times a week to go on walks. Should we keep doing that?"

"You can. Walking has nothing but benefits for him. Do you have any pictures that he likes? I'll turn it into a personalized placemat."

"I'll email them to you."

"There's a living room concert with tasty snacks every Friday afternoon."

"That's nice. He'll probably refuse to listen to the music at first. My father always needs a bit of encouragement."

"We're used to it. What's your father's favorite dish? We'll prepare a personalized menu for him every week."

Thanks to the new assisted living home, I can be a carefree daughter again. I'm still a bit suspicious though. Whenever I get a rare picture of my father on a walk or on a bicycle, I wonder how often they really do these things with him.

Differences

A month after the move, I'm having a drink with a daughter of a resident of the previous assisted living home. She's curious.

"Do you notice any differences between the two places?"

"The most touching thing to me is that we were given a key to the front door on day one, and we were told that we can visit my father anytime. I can be a daughter again and not feel like a visitor. I no longer have to ring the doorbell and wait for a caregiver to come. When my father and I return from a walk, I open the front door with a key. It makes him feel safe."

"How's the care?" the intrigued daughter probes.

"They take incredibly good care of my father. He looks good every day and is served fresh, healthy meals. I can see that he's happy. The caregivers are kind and caring. I do have less contact with other relatives, but I don't mind. I can now focus on my father when I'm there."

"Do you have any points of criticism?"

"Of course, some things could improve. Not everyone is equally well-trained." I tell her about the incident of a caregiver who tried to comfort my father by saying this is his home, while he wanted to go home. My father got angry and the caregiver continued to try to convince him. Luckily, I was able to calm him down by saying that we're just here for a cup of coffee.

"But they do pay more attention to training their staff here. They work with a dementia coach who provides them with guidance on the job."

The daughter's interrogation continues, "What clothes do the caregivers wear at your nursing home?"

"Not their own clothes, like they do at yours. At this nursing home, the caregivers wear a recognizable uniform. I prefer the former. You don't walk around the house in a uniform either." "I agree. It's not a hotel." "Exactly. They like to put paper coasters with the name of the assisted living home on my father's table. I throw them away. It confuses him."

"How do they address the residents?"

"Apparently, there are rules here. In his own room, they call him by his first name. In the hallway, it's Sir or Ma'am. This is based on the idea that the resident's room is their home, and the hallway is outside. I prefer it the way the other nursing home does it, always using their first name. Just like back home."

"Are you happy about the decision to move?" the daughter finally asks.

"I'm ecstatic. And pleased to see my father adjust so quickly."

A week later, a caregiver from the previous home visits my father. I wait for her by the front door. We're glad to see each other and I let her in.

"Oh, look, they've got digital photo frames with alternating photos. Did you make these too?" she asks.

"No, these were here already."

She checks out the entrance. Not spacious, but homey. We agree on that. The hallway of the first home was remarkably spacious. The residents could take quite a proper walk and it was easy for the caregivers to keep an eye on the residents, since the hallway is closed off by glass walls. The drawback was how sterile it all looked.

I heard someone say, "It's like my mother is living in a funeral home."

"It really feels homey in here," says my father's former caregiver. "The downside seems to be that the residents can't really go for a walk in the hallway though."

"That's true, but when a resident grows restless, a caregiver will take them out for a walk around the picturesque neighborhood."

"That sounds perfect. We'd be walking straight onto a busy street. Here, you find yourself in a cute little town."

We walk over to a quiet spot with an armchair and a fireplace in the hallway. "My father calls this the church. The activities coordinator arranged for him to get a church booklet for a mass with stories and hymns." I tell her how much he enjoys withdrawing here with his pious thoughts. He hasn't been too big on religion in the past decades, but the church played an important role in his youth.

We walk to my father's room, where his former caregiver greets him with:

"Hey, neighbor."

At the previous nursing home, my father always used to call her neighbor. He laughs with us. In his room, we see a photo album he made with the activities coordinator. "How nice," says the ex-caregiver, as she browses through the album with pictures of my father at the assisted living home. "Do you have any of the albums here from your vacations and the business, Harry? I always loved looking at those with you."

My father looks at me with the question reflected in his eyes.

"Yes, take a look, they're over there," I point at the stack of photo albums I placed here deliberately. After all, any caregiver who looks at these albums with him will get to know my father better.

We take my father out for lunch. It's touching to see how well the two of them still click. After a couple of enjoyable hours, we take my father back to the home. Then, the caregiver and I stroll around together.

"How are things over there? Still under a lot of pressure?" I ask.

"Yes, but it's the same everywhere," she sighs. "Even though there are more volunteers and interns now, new staff needs to be trained, which takes up a lot of our time." We reach the conclusion that a simple A4 sheet listing the most important rules of dealing with residents, might help.

A sheet of paper with rules of conduct on the inside of the staff restroom door. This way, every caregiver is reminded of it daily.

- Take our residents seriously.
- Speak to them, not about them.
- Never contradict them. Go along with people with dementia.
- Distracting is better than explaining everything.
- Give compliments.
- Chat with them about the things you see around you.
- They aren't stupid and sense a great deal.
- Each resident has their own fascinating life story.

Both assisted living homes are private institutions. The second nursing home is a little more expensive, though. But in return, my father gets a more spacious room with a terrace and fresh, healthy food. In the first assisted living home, they would get meals delivered twice a week and reheat them in the microwave daily. A caregiver even told me they were buying canned soup.

Furthermore, I doubt that my father was getting enough to drink. It's quite a difference whether the amount you pay for your father's care goes to a party that claims to want to become the largest care organization in Europe versus an organization that operates two branches. My sense is that with the former, the money is also put towards opening new branches and not always to the care of current residents. I'm glad that my father now lives in a relatively small assisted living home, where the director considers care to be his mission as opposed to large care organizations, which see care as a business.

50 years

After a pleasant birthday lunch with my brother, I drive on to my father's care home. First, I buy a bottle of cognac and a card at the liquor store. My brother plans to visit my father tonight.

"Hey Dad, are you enjoying your newspaper?" I ask as I walk into his room.

"Hey kid, how nice to see you. How did you know I'm here?" "I always know where to find you."

"What are you holding? A present?" "Yes, for your son. It's his birthday today." "It's his birthday? What date is it?" "December 22."

"Darn. I didn't get him a present."

"I took care of it. This is your gift to him, a bottle of cognac."

"What? A bottle of booze? That's no gift for a child."

"Don't worry about it, Dad. He wanted that bottle."

"I don't care what he wants. This is no good."

"You're right Dad, would you like to write something on this card for your son?"

"Why?"

"It's his birthday, remember?"

"It's my youngest son's birthday?"

"Yes, hence the gift and card."

I manage to get it done. The birthday card receives a nice birthday wish. The door opens. Earlier than expected, my brother walks in with a box of pastries and a chocolate car with the number 50 on it. He gives the chocolate car to my father. I start to sing a birthday song. My father thinks it's his birthday.

"No, Dad. It's my birthday."

"You? How old are you?"

"50."

"50? You're lying."

I can see the confusion in my father's eyes. I realize we should've done this differently. Perhaps it would've been better if I had entered with the bottle of booze in a grocery bag and only had my father write the birthday card in advance. I could've handed to my father the gift and his written birthday card as my brother entered the room. And my brother could've brought a chocolate car, without the number 50 on it. Why should my father be confronted with the fact that his son is turning fifty? To him, his youngest isn't even an adult yet.

Flowers

A week later, I walk into my father's room with a bunch of flowers.

"Those are some gorgeous flowers you've got there."

"They're for you."

"How about Mom? She loves flowers too."

"Sure, for Mom as well."

"Beautiful. Elsa will love these. She'll be back from the grocery store soon."

My mother passed away a year ago now. Several bunches of fake flowers cheer up my father's room. I'm not into fake flowers myself, but he can't really tell the difference anymore. I move a vase of plastic flowers from his table to his closet.

"No! Those flowers are still good. Why would you put them away?"

"To put these fresh ones on the table. They smell so nice. Here, smell them."

"They may smell nice, but I like the other flowers better."

I wonder if the fake flowers might suffice. It'd save me a weekly investment in fresh flowers. I decide to keep surprising him with a fresh bouquet every week. The ritual alone is already worth it. Together we put the flowers in a vase, and as we arrange a fresh bunch of colorful gems of nature, he sits in his chair and sighs:

"Elsa will love these."

Personal Chat Cards

Good conversations with my father occur when I enter the brain room he happens to be in. It comes naturally to me because I know him through and through. This is why it's useful for the caregivers to know the life story of their residents. It helps them take care of them and talk to them. It's a good idea to have these stories written down, since there is a lot of staff turnover and it's difficult to remember all the stories. For this reason, the first home had a life story book for each resident. This was filled in by the resident's loved ones. To equip the caregivers with even more conversation starters, I made personal chat cards. If they have time for a chat with my dad, these cards help them do it more effectively, making it easier for nice conversations to happen. Some examples of my father's chat cards:

<u>Birds</u>

Background:
Harry loves birds, hence the bird feeder outside his window. When he starts to talk about birds, he will definitely have more to tell, especially about great tits, siskins and his favorite bird: the goldfinch. He used to have aviaries, always with at least one quail.

Comments you can make:

It's always nice to have a bird feeder in the garden.

Questions you can ask:

What bird really strikes you as beautiful?

Which birds do you see often and which ones are less common?

Have you ever had an aviary?

Brooms

Background:

Harry used to run the family business. His grandfather once started a factory that made brushes, which grew into a wholesale business in brushes, painting and cleaning supplies.

Comments you can make:

I need to sweep my patio, but I don't know which broom to use.

Questions you can ask:

What types of fibers are there for brooms?

What is a coconut hair broom used for?

What is a scrub brush made of?

How are brooms made?

Did you used to make them all in-house at the factory?

Escaped 3

One morning at breakfast, I open the care file app of my father's assisted living home. I can barely suppress my smile as I read it, though the tragedy of it doesn't escape me.

Harry exited the front door through the garden gate and walked straight into the town. He has returned safely. Please be careful to keep the gate closed.

I read posts like this with some regularity. My mischievous father, the rebel who can't be told what to do, is still present.

My Head is Full of Index Cards

Unexpected things always happen during my visits to my father, either because he wants to go home or doesn't want me to leave. In my head I have a big box full of index cards with various responses. Every time I say goodbye, for example, I use the same card.

"Dad, I'm going out for some groceries."

"Why? That's not necessary, is it?"

"We need groceries for dinner later."

"I'll go with you."

"No, why don't you stay and enjoy your newspaper, Dad. I need to rush my way through the supermarket and it's busy there at this hour. I'll be back soon."

"Do come back. Do you have any cash?"

"Yes, don't worry about it. See you soon, dear."

I give him a pat on the head and walk out of the room, leaving him satisfied with his newspaper. I go home.

I didn't come up with this response card in one go. It improved over time. I started by saying I was going out for groceries. At first, that was enough, and he accepted it, until my father once surprised me by saying he was eager to come along, despite the fact that he doesn't like getting groceries at all. Then, I figured that if I paint a picture of a very busy store, he'll surely pass. I was right.

Another card from my response card index is the following: After a walk, we return to the street that the assisted living home is on.

"Look, we're home."

"Home? I don't live here."

"Yes, you do."

This is where my father refuses to go inside. I've learned to play the following card:

"I need to pick something up here."

"What do you need to pick up?"

"Something important for work. Will you come with me? I'd like that."

I stick the key into the keyhole of the front door of the assisted living home.

"You've got the key?"

"Of course I've got the key. They know me."

We enter together. At first, he doesn't recognize anything, but I see the first signs of recognition in his eyes as he walks through the front door. The recognition is complete when he enters his own room. I can see he feels at home, most of the time. Sometimes, there's another card I need to pull out.

"Hey, our furniture is here. That's strange." I ignore his comment and say:

"Let's have some tea first. Here's your newspaper. Take a seat."

I can see him settle in as he reads his paper in his familiar chair with a cup of tea, and it's now safe to say I'm going out for some groceries.

Once I deploy a card for the first time, it's always a matter of wait and see if it'll work. If my response works, I'll play that card more often. If not, I'll adjust it or come up with a different response. Taking away his driver's license and my story about the test due to the many accidents with cyclists was one of those initial cards. It didn't work. But when I adjusted my story to a temporary driving prohibition due to an expired license, it worked much better. Now, this card doesn't work anymore. When my father wants to go for a drive, all I need to say is: "Today I'm driving. I like to drive. Especially with you next to me."

It gives me peace of mind to be better prepared for potential situations, which is something my father clearly senses.

Another card I like to use when I want to take my father out for lunch is:

"We can't eat here. Elsa is cooking for us," my father will protest.

"Elsa is out with the neighbor," I explain.

"She never mentioned that to me. Are you sure?"

"Yes, I'm sure. She told me. They love hanging out together."

"That's true. They're like two peas in a pod. It's good that she's having a good time." My gaze wanders up. Neither my mother nor the neighbor are alive anymore.

Visit

My son, now fourteen, joins me today to visit his grandfather. I can see my father thinking while his grandson explains who he is. Over tea, my father asks him three times, "What grade are you in again?"

"Ninth grade, Grandpa," he replies patiently.

My father can't believe how big his grandson is. I realize that I have yet to find a solution for this situation. I know my father still sees him as a little boy, and at the same time I'm confronting him with a grandson who is drawing ever closer to adulthood.

A bit later, we're sitting on the terrace of a pancake restaurant. We just enjoyed a nice lunch on the waterfront. I'm surprised to see my father pull out his wallet. He wants to pay, something he used to do all the time. He's been allowing me to treat him lately. But not today.

"Oh boy, I don't think it's enough to pay for lunch," he says when he sees the fifty euros in his wallet. I decide to put some more money in his wallet from now on.

On the way home, my son asks, "Grandpa thinks Grandma Elsa is still alive, doesn't he?"

"Yes, don't you think there's something really beautiful about that? As far as he's concerned, his wife is still alive and well. How does it make you feel when Grandpa talks about Grandma as if she's still alive? Is it hard for you?"

"No, you?"

"No, but I must admit that I do feel a hint of sadness whenever he talks about her. It'd be so nice to still have her around."

Someone Else

I turn the key in the front door of the assisted living home and step inside. My father meets me in the hallway. "Hey Ria, what are you doing here?"

"I've come to visit you."

"Aren't you supposed to be watching Dianca?"

"You know I always take very good care of the sweetest girl in the world. She's upstairs."

"Good. Is she sleeping?"

"Yes, she's resting. I think you have a lovely daughter."

"I do too. She's kind and such a cute girl."

My father mistakes me for his sister Ria, which isn't surprising since I do look a lot like she used to. Normally, I greet my father with: "Hi Dad, your daughter Dianca is here to visit you." It might help him recognize me. But this time, I let it be. It makes me happy that he calls me a sweet and cute girl and is clearly concerned about me. We go to his room together and put the flowers in a vase. He looks at me and says, "Glad you're here, kid."

I place the cookies in a glass cookie jar and the chocolates in a glass dish. My father can see what's inside. Yet, he doesn't usually take anything, at least not without asking. His mother always made him ask before taking anything.

"Did your mother have a cookie jar?" I ask.

"We had a bowl just like the one on the table."

"Did you ever steal a cookie?"

"I'm too scared. Lifting the glass lid makes so much noise."

I realize that if my father doesn't do something, or refuses to do something, I need to carefully consider why he doesn't. I label the sealed glass jars with the text: for Harry. The following week, the jars are less full.

My now seventeen year old daughter asks me after a visit to her grandpa: "Mom, don't you mind that Grandpa mistakes me for you and you for Grandma?"

"Not at all, as long as he feels comfortable around us."

I often find myself explaining to others why I visit my father every week.

"You have to drive an hour and a half each way to visit your father. Why do you do it? He doesn't remember anyway, does he?"

"His smile when I walk in is priceless. It feels good that we can still enjoy our time together."

"So, you do it for your own sake, right? Your father doesn't remember anything."

"I do it for my father too. He lights up when we're outside, having lunch together."

Foggy Future

I notice my father's decline. His walk is becoming more difficult, he's been having all kinds of aches everywhere, and is becoming increasingly withdrawn. When I ask him a question, it takes more time for him to respond. Whenever we go out for lunch, I'll seek out a busy spot now more than ever. I notice a construction site at a restaurant. It fascinates my father. We spend hours sitting there, quietly watching the excavators.

Once winter has passed, I take my father to the construction site, which has now been replaced by a large new building. The restaurant owner greets us enthusiastically and we chat about the construction. My father enthusiastically tries to join the conversation, but the restaurateur walks away. It's painful to watch. I often notice my father being ignored. It's rare for someone to try and engage with him and share a laugh. Society still has a lot to learn when it comes to accepting and dealing with dementia.

I try to ease the pain: "He had to answer the phone. He'll be back soon." When I struggle to connect with him, I place my hands on his knee, and he gives me a smile. As long as he enjoys himself and seems content, it feels right. Step by step, we face the foggy future together.

I catch your gaze
So empty, I sigh

Once again, I attempt
To go to your present: the past

You tell a story all your own
Full of familiar language and tone

I like to listen
And inquire

You smile
Your eyes soften

You speak with an aura of bliss
Little moments of happiness

What I Learned About Dementia

I listed the lessons I've learned, and those shared with me by other loved ones, in the hope that it may help other family caregivers.

At Home

Situations

Going Out Alone

Whenever my father had gone out alone, we made sure:

to inform whoever he thought he was going to visit,

there was a GPS tracker and a note with my contact information in my father's pocket.

It's best to give them a pre-programmed cellphone to bring with them, but we never managed to do it. My father resisted the idea of being reachable all the time.

Home Alone

My mother would put a note on the table saying where she'd be. To avoid writing the same thing over and over again, she kept the written notes in a tin. I'd call my father whenever I knew my mother wasn't home. I'd quickly figure out if he knew where she was or if he was disoriented. If I'd find him disoriented, I'd call again 15 minutes later. This would often have a reassuring effect.

By the time the disease had progressed, we made sure to hire a sitter. My father refused to accept it, until the sitter started cleaning. Whenever she was there, my father was able do his own thing while the sitter kept an eye on him.

Going out together

I still take my father out a lot. Whenever he needs to go to the bathroom at a restaurant, I'll walk with him. I'll tell him I need to go too, otherwise he won't let me come. I'll wait in front of the men's room. He smiles at me as he comes out of the bathroom, and I know he's happy to see me.

Whenever I leave our table to go pay inside, I give my father the task of keeping a close eye on my handbag. He'll remain seated in his chair with the bag clasped in his hands.

Outsiders don't always notice that my father has dementia, which can be problematic. It can create confusion, for instance in a store. I've carry a note that says, "My father has dementia." I'd hold it up behind his back to help people understand.

Taking Away the Driver's License

I made up a story to get my father to stop driving his car. Emphasizing that his driver's license was gone temporarily because it had expired, worked well. A relative told me that he parked the car out of his father's sight. This was enough to prevent his father from wanting to drive again.

Delusion

At times my father became delusional. Correcting him wasn't helpful. I found that I was able to change the subject quite quickly, as long as I said that I believe him and will help him find a solution.

Celebrations with Dementia

We noticed that involving my father in everything was becoming increasingly counterproductive. We decided to stop telling him anything about our plans and organized surprise parties and surprise vacations instead. Others have told me that it actually helps to diligently inform their loved ones. One son told me that he writes up a comprehensive document on the upcoming vacation a month in advance, so his father can rejoice over and over again.

Passing of a Loved One

In hindsight, I made a big mistake by taking my father to my mother's funeral. Why did we do that? For our own benefit? For the outside world? Because my mother would've wanted us to? In any case, I caused him a lot of grief that day. Mourning takes time, which he doesn't have because he keeps forgetting. I'll tell him again, and he'll start mourning again. We decided to stop confronting my father with the fact that his wife has passed away. In his world, his wife is alive and well.

Afternoon Restlessness

My father became especially restless in the afternoon. I discovered that this had to do with the natural light that starts diminishing around that time. My father would start packing all kinds of things into his car. He thought he was at a vacation home and wanted to go to his parents' house. It would help to have a walking companion come over or distract him with videos. It also helped to have him drink less coffee or give him decaffeinated coffee during the day. Every afternoon was a quest for what worked best. Later on, he was given Risperidone by the doctor to help with the restlessness. The medication helped for a while.

Waking Up in the Middle of the night

My father would regularly wake up at night, get out of bed and start getting dressed. In most cases, my mother managed to stop him by showing him that it was dark outside and pointing to the clock. Another relative told me that he felt he had made the following mistake. His mother lived alone and would become restless at night. To make sure she wouldn't walk off, he'd lock all the doors and hide the keys. He'd feel guilty about it afterwards. He found her completely disoriented in the living room one morning. It was time for her to move to an assisted living home.

Preparing for Care

I had prepared myself for the help I might have to get for my parents. My mother kept refusing, while I had prepared for all the possible scenarios with the corresponding solutions. This included contact details of assistance agencies that I had already contacted, ranging from home care organizations to private nurses and sitters.

I also requested some quotations for assisted living homes. It gave me peace of mind. When my father suddenly deteriorated very rapidly and my mother could no longer cope with caring for him, my preparation allowed me to move quickly. In hindsight, I didn't start looking for assisted living homes in time and should've done a more thorough job. Walk into a nursing home unexpectedly. Get a sense of the atmosphere. The beautifully designed brochures promise freshly made meals and regular activities, but is it true? Take a look around dinner time or volunteer to help out for a day.

Telling the Grandchildren

I explained to my children (then nine and twelve years old) that their grandpa wasn't well. I told them that the wiring in his brain is broken and the body can't repair it anymore. His forgetfulness and bad temper are consequences of that.

Interaction

Distraction

Distraction really works. When a conversation isn't going in the direction I want it to go, there's always a painting or a bird somewhere that I can use to distract him.

Compliments

My father lights up when I give him a compliment. It puts him in a good mood.

Dodging the Truth

I do lie to my father at times, but I never mislead him. I do everything for his own good. I change the facts to reassure him. I discovered that I could avoid painful truths. If you can't lie outright, just look for alternative words.

Brain Rooms

I visualize my father's brain as a building full of rooms with memories. His brain rooms are valuable treasures to him. He lives in them and occasionally moves to another room. When visiting my father, I try to discover which room he's in. Is it that of his early childhood, his youth or is he in the room of his adult self? It always takes some searching to find an open door. Within the walls of this room, I can start a conversation and even ask questions that he will answer. By going along with him, I see that he feels heard and feels that I take him seriously.

My Head is Full of Index Cards

I have a box full of index cards in my head with self-created responses that I can use at unexpected moments. At any time, I can draw a card that seems appropriate for the situation and that can help distract and direct my father to a situation where he feels safe. I often use the same card for similar situations.

Harmonious Interaction

I discover that force never works. We explain things clearly, show my father what's going to happen and reassure him. When my father talks to me, I have to be patient. He now has a harder time finding words and needs time. If I correct him or contradict him, it can ruin the atmosphere. I learn that I can chat with him about things we can both observe. We can just share the moment together by keeping it nice and simple.

Learning

It's a misconception that people with dementia can no longer learn anything. I teach my father to operate the complicated on/off switch on a new lamp just by demonstrating it a few times.

Entertainment

My father is calmer when stimulated. It doesn't have to involve any extravagant activities. I recently read somewhere that people with dementia remain stable in their disease progression when they receive enough stimulation. At home, we made sure his daytime activities remained meaningful through:

Daily Chores

My father would cut the grass, carry groceries from the car and feed the animals. When mowing the lawn, he'd feel useful, and my mother would have some time to herself.

Newspapers or Puzzle Books

My father loves to read newspapers. We subscribed him to three papers. Another relative told me that her father-in-law liked to do puzzles. They purchased piles of booklets full of puzzles.

A Walking Companion

We found a walking companion. They sacrificed their own time to walk with my father. We thought it made sense to pay them for their service. It also made it easier for my mother to ask them more frequently. Another relative told me that she pays her mother's neighbors to keep an eye on her and to cook for her mother. As a result, her mother can continue to live at home without the need for home care.

Videos on a Laptop

My father made many videos in his life. I copied them onto a laptop. My father can really enjoy watching his own camera work. YouTube videos of Laurel and Hardy, for example, make for a good diversion as well.

Music

My father is not much of a music buff, but another relative told me that her mother used to love The Beatles. All she had to do to put a smile on her mother's face was put on some of their music. Others told me their parents love to dance to music they know.

Personal Affairs

Living Will

A living will describes who gets authority over your assets and care, should you become incapacitated. It has te be created before dementia gets diagnosed.

We are glad we created a living will at the time. Now that my mother has passed away, my brothers and I can manage my father's affairs without the intervention of a judge.

Changing contact information

We registered my phone number with the hospital, the doctor and other important contacts, and had my parents' landline deleted from their systems. It would cause problems if my father would pick up the phone and forgot to pass on a message.

Help

Alarm Button at Home

We requested an alarm button from a home care agency. It made me feel reassured that my mother always had the button nearby as a kind of escape. If she pressed the button, a home care worker would try to contact her. If that didn't work, they'd be at her door within 15 minutes.

Various Websites

I'd show my mother educational websites and sign her up for email newsletters about dementia. Reading stories of others in similar situations would give us strength.

Books About Dementia

Reading books about dementia helped me understand what the disease does to my father's brain. Reading recognizable stories gives me strength, I can pick up tips here and there that I can try and put into practice. There are many wonderful and informative books about dementia out there.

The Doctor

My parents' doctor was an important source of support for me. Even though I was not his patient, he was always welcoming whenever I had questions about my parents. I only visited him a few times. It's nice to know that I can turn to him.

Sitter

My mother engaged a sitter. But as soon as she'd get back home, her day would be all about caring for my father. We'd organize a weekend or a week vacation with my parents on a regular basis. Having everyone together like that allowed us to share the load of caring for him.

Aids

Hearing Impaired

Hearing aids were helpful to my father for a while. It's best to purchase custom hearing aids, but they are expensive. Many people with dementia don't want to wear them. Be sure to test this in advance. We turned on the subtitles on my father's television. Headphones helped as well, although my father wouldn't always want to put them on.

Visually Impaired

A simple TV remote with large buttons worked well for my father. Another relative told me that he bought a magnifying glass and a reading ruler with a magnifying glass for his mother, who had trouble reading. It helped his mother enjoy her magazines again.

Deteriorating Motor Skills

I noticed that my father stopped opening his cookie jars. I now put cookies and chocolates in glass jars. The glass lid is easier to lift, and my father can see what's inside. Another relative told me that she would have bought a walker much earlier if she had known that her mother still enjoyed walking so much. You can even get one secondhand for a modest amount.

No Sense of Time

My father lost track of the days. We purchased a clearly readable clock with a day indicator.

Assisted Living

Getting to Know My Father

Life story book

The first nursing home gave us a life story book, asking us to fill in the questions in the book. Caregivers told us that, unfortunately, not all of them read the book. Plus, they found it quite difficult to remember all the residents' backgrounds.

Personal Care Document

When my father moved to another nursing home, I wrote up my own personal care document, describing briefly the most important care issues.

Personal Chat Cards

It's easy for me to enter my father's open brain rooms, since I know his life story. To help the caregivers, I created a set of personal chat cards. Should they have time to talk to my father, it'll be easier to have a nice conversation this way.

Communication at an Assisted Living Home

Triangle

Care for people with dementia should be based on the triangle of residents, care teams and relatives. In my experience, there is room for improvement in this regard. Caregivers: Do enlist the help of loved ones. They will often help, and go about it in a loving way. It makes a difference, especially today, when almost every assisted living home is understaffed.

Conversations between Caregivers and Relatives

It's been my experience that caregivers often don't have much time to talk to relatives. They'll usually only mention a few things in passivy during my visits to my father. If someone has dementia it is important to talk with them and not about them. My father is hard of hearing and doesn't follow all the conversations well. While talking to a caregiver, I often make eye contact with my father or indicate that I'll explain everything to him later. I notice that he's okay with that.

Communication with Relatives

In both assisted living homes, I should've been more diligent about finding out what communication channels are being used. In the first home, my mother had been sending messages to the care team through the electronic care record system for six months. These messages were never read. In the second home, my messages first failed to arrive at first as well. Upon inquiry, I was told that a setting in the electronic care system needed to be changed. What is missing at the second home, is a monthly newsletter with updates on things like activities, caregivers and other developments. They do organize however an annual barbecue and a concert for the residents and their loved ones. What very helpful is that they hire a dementia coach almost every year to spend an evening with the relatives in order to help them to navigate of dementia.

Communication with Residents

One assisted living home had put up a sheet with communication rules on the inside of the restroom door.

It helped temporary staff or new employees to quickly learn and understand the rules, as well as how to interact with people with dementia.

- Take our residents seriously.
- Talk to them, not about them.
- Never contradict them. Go along with people with dementia.
- Distracting is better than explaining everything.

- Give compliments.
- Chat with them about the things you see around you.
- People with dementia aren't stupid and sense a great deal.
- Each resident has their own fascinating life story.

Client Council

I became a member of the client council. As a result, my contact with the caregivers increased, as did my knowledge about the care choices being made at the care organization. Most assisted living homes have a family or client council.

Situations

Parties

Celebrating my father's birthday has become a challenge since he moved into the assisted living home. It pains me to watch his confusion upon seeing decorations or getting birthday cards with his age; in his world, he's much younger. We once tried spreading out the visits throughout his birthday, which he thoroughly enjoyed. But when he turned eighty, we wanted the whole family to celebrate together, with his children and grandkids. We would actively try to keep him involved in our conversations through out the day. The celebration began in my brother's yard, and given my father's cheerful mood, we ventured take him to a restaurant. He kept going surprisingly well, and when I read that he had slept through the night in his care file the next day, I realized that we shouldn't shield him too much. It would rob him of some wonderful moments.

Difficulty Saying Goodbye

My mother always struggled to say goodbye to my father after visits. A caregiver picked up my father and invited him to dinner in the sunroom. He asked why my mother wasn't coming and accepted the excuse that she had to go get some dessert. My mother watched as the caregiver took him to the dining room, cheerful as ever.

My Father Doesn't Recognize Me

I always greet my father when I enter his room with: "Hi, Dad, don't be alarmed. It's me, Dianca."

Chances are, he'll know who I am. If he still doesn't recognize me, I drop it for a while. He'll usually know who I am after a couple of minutes.

Moving

We used his own familiar furniture from the past when decorating my father's room at the assisted living home.

A caregiver told me she really likes that. Not just because it makes my father feel at home, but also because it informs her, as his caregiver, what his home used to look like.

Interaction

Aggressive or Angry

My father gets angry sometimes when caregivers try to help him in the morning. Other relatives regularly tell me that their parent will suddenly show aggressive or angry behavior. By now, I know that angry behavior has to come from somewhere. Don't laugh at it; instead, look for the cause. Often, someone with dementia just wants to communicate something. It's the only way fort hem to let you know about their discontent.

Record Keeping

Another relative gave me a good piece of advice. He and his relatives keep a notebook in which they write down what makes their mother happy. This allows them to try and put a smile on her face every day.

Entertainment

Personal Activity Program

We set up our own activity program, entertaining my father at least five times a week. We'll take him for a walk, go out to have some lunch together or play a game in his room. This is to ensure that he gets enough distraction and we're not dependent on understaffed caregivers. Consider any activity organized by the nursing home as a nice extra.

Lunch

I like to take my father out for lunch. I make sure there's always something going on where we eat, such as a view of a busy square or even a construction site. He'll be watching closely everything that's going on around him with a content look in his eyes.

My brothers and I agreed that if someone takes my father out, the bill can be paid from my father's own bank account. This allows my father to treat his grandson to dinner, just like he used to.

Newspapers

We register my father's three newspaper subscriptions to the nursing home. We agreed with the caregivers that they will hand them out throughout the day, so my father gets to enjoy his daily newspapers all day long and has a moment of contact with the caregiver when the paper is delivered.

Refilling the Bird Feeder

At the first assisted living home, they hardly ever took my father out for a walk. We provided two bird feeders for the garden and bought food for the birds. My father enjoyed refilling the feeders together with a caregiver. This provided him with much needed distraction while getting a little exercise at the same time.

Display Cabinets

At the first nursing home, caregivers had installed two display cabinets and asked relatives to fill them with items from the past. One cabinet was filled with old model cars, for instance. My father spent hours looking at them from a chair that was placed in front of the display.

Digital Photo Frame

There is a digital photo frame filled with nature pictures on the service counter at my father's assisted living home. It always catches the attention of some of the residents.

A Box with Games

My mother put a box with games under my father's bed. I pull out a game every now and then. My father was never into games, but he really seems to enjoy them these days.

Photo albums

I have made photo albums full of pictures of past vacations, celebrations, or births. It's always fun for yourself or a caregiver to flip through an album with your loved one. A further benefit for the caregiver is that they get to know your loved one that much better.

Epilogue

People with dementia all have their own stories. They've had a full life. They've worked hard, cared for their own parents and children, and they have their own strong opinions. They were looked up to, or deeply loved in their neighborhood. Since they've entered this phase of their lives, they've been vulnerable. We don't know exactly what's going on inside their heads. How lonely must that be? We must try to gain access to the world of people with dementia, to help them and embrace them as who they are now.

Informal caregivers work tirelessly to surround their relative with love. They sacrifice some of their own freedom out of a sense of duty and respect for who their loved one once was. I recognize this in myself. The process of my father's illness is a struggle for me. Frustration and sadness alternate with my own insecurity as the overtone. Am I doing it right? What else can I do to increase the joy in his life? These are the questions that occupy my thoughts every day. I feel responsible for his well-being, especially now that my mother has passed away. I'm privileged that my father is now living in a good assisted living home. It gives me peace of mind.

I've written down my own learning process for others who also have increasing difficulty understanding their loved one. I hope for this book to contribute to a little more insight into dementia. My biggest lesson was learning to get a better feel for my father. I understand his instruction manual better and see the person he is now, mixed with the person he once was. Every week, I experience moments with him that I enjoy. I wish these moments of happiness for everyone who is dealing with dementia.

My father's illness is always changing. For me it is a a continuous process of adjusting and looking for the best way to interact. If you're interested in the progress of my dementia learning process, please visit www.DiancaSchussler.com I'd love to meet you there.